Arts Therapies in Schools

of related interest

Meditation and Movement
Structured Therapeutic Activity Sessions
G. Rosser
ISBN 978 1 84905 018 0

Using Expressive Arts to Work with Mind, Body and Emotions
Theory and Practice
Mark Pearson and Helen Wilson
ISBN 978 1 84905 031 9

Focusing-Oriented Art Therapy
Accessing the Body's Wisdom and Creative Intelligence
Laury Rappaport
ISBN 978 1 84310 760 6

Art as an Early Intervention Tool for Children with Autism
Nicole Martin
ISBN 978 1 84905 807 0

Art Therapy Techniques and Applications
Susan I. Buchalter
ISBN 978 1 84905 806 3

Breath in Action
The Art of Breath in Vocal and Holistic Practice
Edited by Jane Boston and Rena Cook
ISBN 978 1 84310 942 6

Creative Coping Skills for Children
Emotional Support through Arts and Crafts Activities
Bonnie Thomas
Illustrated by Bonnie Thomas
ISBN 978 1 84310 921 1

Classroom Tales
Using Storytelling to Build Emotional, Social and Academic Skills across the Primary Curriculum
Jennifer M. Fox Eades
ISBN 978 1 84310 304 2

Arts Therapies in Schools

Research and Practice

Edited by Vicky Karkou

Jessica Kingsley Publishers
London and Philadelphia

The image for the cover titled 'footballers' is based on a drawing by 'Alistair', 6 year old boy attending art therapy (see chapter 9). Produced with permission.

First published in 2010
by Jessica Kingsley Publishers
116 Pentonville Road
London N1 9JB, UK
and
400 Market Street, Suite 400
Philadelphia, PA 19106, USA

www.jkp.com

Library of Congress Cataloging in Publication Data

Arts therapies in schools : research and practice / edited by Vicky Karkou.
p. cm.
Includes bibliographical references and index.
ISBN 978-1-84310-633-3 (pb : alk. paper) 1. Art therapy for children. 2. School psychology. 3. School children--Mental health services. I. Karkou, Vassiliki.
LB3430.A78 2010
371.7'13--dc22
2009020001

British Library Cataloguing in Publication Data

A CIP catalogue record for this book is available from the British Library

ISBN 978 1 84310 633 3

Printed and bound in Great Britain by
MPG Books Limited, Cornwall

To my family, who taught me the value of learning and the need to learn 'well'.

Contents

INTRODUCTION 9
Vicky Karkou, Queen Margaret University, Edinburgh, Scotland

Part I: Mainstream Schools ***25***

1. From the Dance Studio to the Classroom: Translating the Clinical Dance Movement Psychotherapy Experience into a School Context 27
Suzi Tortora, Dance/Movement Psychotherapist, Dancing Dialogue, New York, United States

2. PEACE through Dance/Movement Therapy: The Development and Evaluation of a Violence Prevention Programme in an Elementary School 43
Lynn Koshland, Dance/Movement Therapist and Social Worker, Salt Lake City, Utah, United States

3. Finding a Way Out of the Labyrinth through Dance Movement Psychotherapy: Collaborative Work in a Mental Health Promotion Programme for Secondary Schools 59
Vicky Karkou, Ailsa Fullarton, Art Therapist, Glasgow, Scotland; and Susan Scarth, Queen Margaret University, Edinburgh, Scotland

4. Making Space Inside: The Experience of Dramatherapy within a School-based Student Support Unit 85
Jo Christensen, Dramatherapist, Cornwall, England

5. Solution-focused Brief Dramatherapy Group Work: Working with Children in Mainstream Education in Sri Lanka 97
Genevieve Smyth, Dramatherapist, Edinburgh, Scotland

6. The Searching Drama of Disaffection: Dramatherapy Groups in a Whole-school Context 114
Toby Quibell, Dramatherapist, Learning Challenge, Northumberland, England

7. Educational Music Therapy: Theoretical Foundations Explored in Time-limited Group Work Projects with Children 129
Emma Pethybridge, Music Therapist, Herdmanflat Hospital, Haddington, Scotland, and James Robertson, Queen Margaret University, Edinburgh, Scotland

8. Art Therapy in Education for Children with Specific Learning Difficulties Who Have Experienced Stress and/or Trauma 145
Unnur Ottarsdottir, the Reykjavik Academy and Art Therapy Studio, Iceland

9. 'Give Me Some Paper': The Role of Image-making as a Stabilizing Force for a Child in Transition 161
Frances Prokofiev, Art Therapist, London, England

Part II: Special Schools ***177***

10. 'I Am Here to Move and Dance with You': Dance Movement Therapy with Children with Autism Spectrum Disorder and Pervasive Developmental Disorders 179
Hilda Wengrower, University of Barcelona, Spain

11. Dramatherapy, Autism and Relationship-building: A Case Study 197
Lynn Tytherleigh, Dramatherapist, England, and Vicky Karkou

12. The Capacity for Imagination: Implications for Working with Children with Autism in Art Therapy 217
Fuyuko Takeda, Art Therapist, England

13. Music Therapy for Children with Autism in an Educational Context 231
Jo Tomlinson, Music Therapist, England

14. Unmasking Hidden Resources: Communication in Children with Severe Developmental Disabilities in Music Therapy 243
Cochavit Elefant, University of Bergen, Norway

15. Facing the Challenge: A Music Therapy Investigation in the Evidence-based Framework 259
Katrina McFerran, University of Melbourne, Australia, and Jennifer Stephenson, Macquarie University, Australia

SUMMARY AND CONCLUSIONS 271
Vicky Karkou

THE CONTRIBUTORS 280

INDEX 284

Introduction

Vicky Karkou

This is a book about arts therapies in schools, encompassing music, art, drama and dance movement psychotherapy,[1] and brings together international contributions dealing with research and practice in the field. The necessity for this book has become apparent through my own engagement in therapy, teaching and research in this area. For many years I found myself being one of the few people researching and publishing on the topic. At the same time I was aware that there were several arts therapists practising in mainstream and special schools. It was therefore clear that work completed in this context was not receiving sufficient attention within English language literature.

As we will see in the sections following, other reasons for publishing this book have been:

- the historical links between arts therapies and arts education
- the belief that work environments can have a major impact upon the practice of arts therapies, such that there is a need to identify useful ways of working within this context

1 'Dance movement psychotherapy' is the new name for the discipline in the UK as agreed by the Association in Dance Movement Psychotherapy UK in June 2009. However, in most other European countries the name of the discipline remains 'dance movement therapy'. In this book, the terms 'dance movement therapy' and 'dance movement *psycho*therapy' will be used interchangeably to refer to the same discipline.

Similar debates can also be found in other disciplines. Art therapy, for example, is also known as 'art psychotherapy'. Both terms are legally protected under the Health Professions Council (HPC). However, in this context, the contributors decided to call their practice 'art therapy' and so this is the term used throughout the book for that particular discipline.

For drama, the British term 'dramatherapy' is used throughout the book instead of the American term 'drama therapy'. The reason for this is, again, the fact that it is the preferred term used by the contributors.

- the fact that there is limited research work completed and reported from this context, and a need to integrate research and practice in appropriate, useful and therapeutically sound ways.

Towards the end of this introduction the reader will also find a broad description of the key features of the book and a brief overview of the chapters included.

HISTORICAL LINKS BETWEEN ARTS THERAPIES AND EDUCATION

Arts therapists have had a lengthy involvement with supporting children and adolescents in school environments. Early accounts of the emergence of the field in the UK, for example, report that a large part of early pioneering work has already begun in schools (Jennings 1987; Payne 1992; Waller 1992; Wigram 1993). The contribution of child-centred education, with its emphasis upon emotional and social development, has enabled the development of arts therapies in this country (Karkou 1999; Karkou and Glasman 2004; Karkou and Sanderson 2000, 2001, 2006). Furthermore, according to Waller (1992), in the early days of the profession arts therapies were seen as a sensitive form of arts teaching. To some extent this view still persists, despite the fact that the two fields are now officially separate. In the UK the introduction of the National Curriculum has been partly responsible for putting an end to the prominence of child-centred education. The attention of arts educators has been shifted from valuing children's psychological well-being (and what was known as the 'emotional curriculum') to a primary concern of developing artistic outcomes. At the same time, arts therapies had begun to evolve as separate professions in terms of setting up associations and training programmes, establishing career structures, and clarifying separate professional identities. Movements towards professionalization have culminated in arts therapies becoming regulated by the Health Professions Council (HPC) as health professions alongside occupational therapy, physiotherapy and speech and language therapy.

The recognition of arts therapies as a health profession implies that the differences between arts education have become even more apparent. Potentially, this has consequences for practice. Some of the most important differences between arts education and arts therapies are discussed by

Karkou and Glasman (2004), Karkou and Sanderson (2006), and are summarized here. Arts education and arts therapies are seen in terms of:

- differences of intention; arts education aims towards aesthetic and artistic outcomes, while arts therapies have a clear psychological intent
- differences of content; arts teaching involves an artistic curriculum, while arts therapists have a therapeutic agenda
- presence or absence of arts instruction; the arts teacher will instruct, while the arts therapist tends not to (unless there is a clear psychological need to do so)
- attention to artistic change; in arts teaching artistic change is seen as important in its own right, while in arts therapies artistic change gives information about associated psychological change.

We can also see differences between the two fields in terms of practical applications, such as the tendency of arts teachers to use open spaces (art or dance studio, gym), while most of the work that arts therapists do is kept within private and confidential spaces. There are also differences in the size of groups. While arts teachers often work with a large number of children, arts therapists tend to work either one-to-one or with small groups.

Further discussion of similarities and differences between arts therapies and arts education can be found in the available literature (see Bunt 1994; Payne 1992; Peter 1998; Sanderson 1996; Warwick 1995; Wengrower 2001; Valente and Fontana 1991).

SCHOOLS AS AN IMPORTANT WORKING ENVIRONMENT FOR ARTS THERAPISTS

Despite growing differences between the two disciplines, schools remain a fairly common working environment for arts therapists. In a UK nationwide survey of practitioners (Karkou 1998; Karkou and Sanderson 2006), education appeared to be the second most frequently reported area of work for arts therapists following work in the health service. Looking at each of the disciplines separately (see Figure i), schools have had a particularly prominent place amongst dance movement psychotherapists and music therapists (less so amongst art therapists).

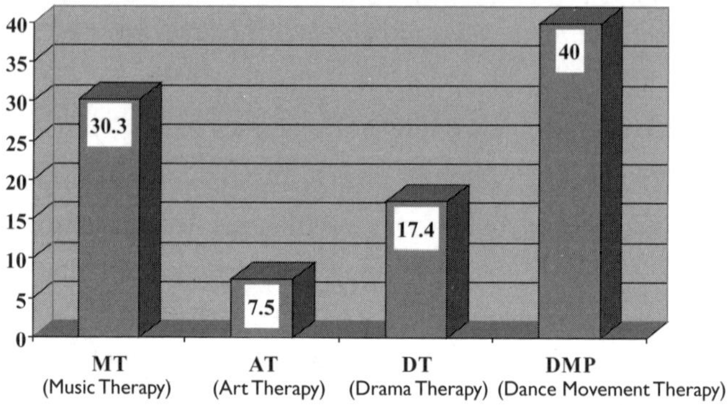

Figure i: Arts therapies in schools in the UK

It is worth noting that a relatively larger proportion of dance movement psychotherapists and music therapists appear to work in education in comparison with arts therapists and dramatherapists. Specific historical and professional developments can account for variations between disciplines. For example, in dance movement psychotherapy there has been an uninterrupted history of employment of practitioners in schools. The contributions of Laban and modern educational dance in the early days of the development of the particular arts therapies discipline, and the prominence of Laban's ideas in current practice, may be associated with the large proportion of dance movement psychotherapists working in schools (40%). Educational dance stemming from Laban (1960) has been widespread in British schools, and is particularly conducive to therapeutic work and the emergence of dance movement psychotherapy as a separate discipline in the UK (Karkou and Sanderson 2000, 2001). The close link between the two disciplines makes it plausible that dance movement psychotherapists working in education are also trained as teachers and are expected to carry out a dual role as teacher and therapist. It is also possible that once registration of dance movement psychotherapy with the HPC is completed (the professional association was accepted for registration with HPC in 2004 and has since been awaiting parliamentary time that will enable the completion of the process), the national picture for this discipline will change, possibly with a number of practitioners shifting from employment in schools to being employed by the NHS.

It is interesting that pioneering work in education has also been reported in art therapy. However, Figure i shows that only a small percentage of art therapists (less than 10%) report employment in schools as their main working environment. Waller (1992) refers to the original alignment of the British Art Therapy Association (BAAT) with the National Union of Teachers (NUT). However, this alliance was subsequently dropped in order to ease off interprofessional conflicts and pursue recognition of the art therapy profession within the National Health Service. It is possible that it was as a result of this decision that the number of art therapists working in schools dropped significantly. A similar situation is witnessed in other European countries too. In Latvia and Russia, for example, a close connection of arts therapies with arts education has been characteristic of the early days of the profession. However, in Latvia, as the profession is currently growing, the link with education is weakening in favour of alliances with the medical profession and the health service (Martinsone, Karkou and Nazarova 2009).

It is likely that the move from education to the health service may be followed by a renewed shift back to working in schools. As the health system changes and principles of community care, multi-sector collaboration and prevention become particularly relevant, working in schools is currently receiving renewed attention and consideration. Education remains the setting where children at risk of developing mental health problems can have their initial contact with responsible adults and qualified professionals. Through this contact, difficulties can be identified early and can be addressed before it becomes necessary to resort to the aid of specialized services outside the school environment. In all cases, it is possible that arts therapists can play a valuable role.

THE IMPACT OF THE SCHOOL ENVIRONMENT UPON ARTS THERAPIES PRACTICE

This book is also founded on the belief that the context can have a major impact upon practice. In previous studies (Karkou 1998; Karkou and Sanderson 2006) it has become apparent that, next to the needs of the client group itself, the type of setting that arts therapists work in plays an important role in the therapeutic orientation of the work. Working with children within this environment is very different from working with children in the health service, within social services or the community. The predominance of learning theory and the need to produce cognitive outcomes and reach achievement targets often sets a very specific perspective through which arts therapists are invited to view the psychological needs of children and adolescents. In most school environments, addressing emotional or social needs is seen as a way of supporting learning, i.e. developing skills and achieving cognitive outcomes.

Arts therapists often have to re-think their practice in order to fit within the overall philosophy of the school and the needs of their clients. For example, arts therapy practice informed by psychodynamic thinking, that has emerged from working with adult mental health clients in the health service, will need to be reconsidered when working with children within a school environment (Karkou and Sanderson 2006). In the UK survey of practitioners completed by Karkou (1998) and published in Karkou and Sanderson (2006), arts therapists working in schools showed a closer affiliation with humanistic ideas. The relevance of this theoretical frame to working in schools can be further explored, alongside the value of psychodynamic/psychoanalytic thinking, developmental work and particular ideas emerging from within the arts therapies disciplines.

RESEARCH IN ARTS THERAPIES PRACTICE IN EDUCATION

There is a growing expectation that the practice of arts therapies will be well informed by research and thoroughly evaluated. Words like 'evidence', 'evidence-based practice', 'practice-based evidence', 'evaluation' and 'research' are frequently used within the health system, at least within a UK context. In recent years, debates regarding the same issues seem to have also extended to school environments. Davies (1999) explains the meaning of 'evidence-based education' (a term first introduced by Hargreaves in 1997 as an adaptation from the more extensively used term 'evidence-based medicine'), while Coe (1999) describes the manifesto for evidence-based education as an important characteristic of contemporary educational practice.

However, if we look at these debates more closely we will see that there is no agreement about what constitutes good research evidence. The hierarchy of evidence that is often associated with effectiveness is presented in Table i.

This way of looking at evidence for arts therapies creates a number of problems. For one thing, the prominence of quantitative evidence and the medical/behavioural ethos of viewing evidence as presented in Table i clashes with the creative content of arts therapies practice. The need to bring the arts to the centre of research studies in arts therapies has been long discussed in the arts therapies literature (e.g. McNiff 1998;

Table i: Hierarchy of evidence

1.	Evidence from meta-analyses or systematic reviews or at least one Randomized Controlled Trial (RCT)
2.	Evidence from at least one controlled study without randomization or one other quasi-experimental study
3.	Evidence from descriptive studies such as comparative studies, correlation studies, case-control series, multiple case studies
4.	Evidence from reports or opinions from expert committees or experience of respected authorities in clinical practice

(adapted from Eccles, Freemantle and Mason 2001)

Wadsworth-Hervey 2000). Furthermore, this particular hierarchy of evidence can often clash with the fact that within arts therapies, and within many other psychotherapeutic interventions, emphasis is placed upon client experiences and internal processes rather than overt and quantifiable behavioural changes (Gilroy 2006; Fonagy *et al.* 2002). Arguments have been put forward about the need for the definition of evidence to include and equally value qualitative and arts-based information. At least the call for qualitative evidence is now considered by the Cochrane Collaboration (2009) with a qualitative research methods group currently in existence. At the same time, there is a need for arts therapists to engage with what *can* be quantified and *can* be measured, especially given the need to improve existing conditions of work and establish new posts within school environments.

On the whole, and despite the evidence that research activity in arts therapies is flourishing (e.g. research registers held with arts therapies professional associations; systematic reviews available from the Cochrane Database of Systematic Reviews), completed research studies regarding work in schools are insufficiently and intermittently documented. Similarly, there is limited information about the therapeutic approaches that are useful for arts therapists working in this environment. Also, there is neither a single book that includes a thorough discussion of the role of arts therapies within school-related policies, and initiatives such as mental health promotion or social inclusion programmes; nor is there a compilation of studies that present research evidence and thus contribute towards well informed and appropriate therapeutic interventions. Existing books look at specific types of arts therapies disciplines (e.g. Heal and Wigram 1993 in music therapy; Bush 1997 and Moriya 2000 in art therapy; Crimmens 2006 and McFarlane 2005 in dramatherapy). This limits the potential to learn from similar practices in the other arts therapies. Other books look at specific symptoms or needs (Evans and Dubowski 2001; Stein-Safran 2002) but often fail to address the fact that arts therapists placed in schools are faced with a wide diversity of children's needs. Finally, existing publications refer to work completed in a particular school in a particular country. This makes it difficult to identify some common themes emerging from working in education across settings and cultures.

A BRIEF DESCRIPTION OF THIS BOOK

This book has been designed to address an apparent gap in the literature and offers a unique first picture of the work of arts therapies in schools. Its key characteristics are:

1. inclusion of examples of work from all four arts therapies (music, art, drama and dance movement psycho/therapy) in both mainstream and special schools
2. reference to working with diverse needs of children that reflect the diversity of needs faced by arts therapists working in schools
3. emphasis placed on research and routine evaluation completed in the field that follow quantitative, qualitative and/or arts-based methodologies
4. inclusion of contributions from a number of different therapists practising in the USA, Australia, Israel, Spain, Norway and Sri Lanka. This gives it an international context, wider than a singular British one.

As a result of its novelty and its wide-ranging content, the book is expected to be of interest not only to arts therapists but also to professionals linked with school education, such as teachers, and arts teachers in particular; teaching assistants; Special Educational Needs Co-ordinators (SENCOs); guidance teachers; educational psychologists; school nurses and counsellors; health professionals; artists working within or out of the schools; and, potentially, parents and parent associations. Furthermore, given the international nature of its contributions, my hope is that arts therapists throughout the world will find the book engaging and useful.

The book is structured in two parts:

- Part I deals with contributions from work completed in mainstream schools.
- Part II includes contributions from arts therapies practice in special schools.

Part I starts with two contributions from the USA in dance movement psychotherapy. First, Suzi Tortora discusses her therapeutic intervention with a child dealing with issues around control and bullying, with the child being the instigator of violent and disruptive behaviour (Chapter 1). Suzi's work takes place in her dance studio, the place where the child comes to see her for two years. The therapeutic intervention is thoroughly evaluated using monitoring forms that include detailed descriptions of the sessions, further analysis of selected events and longitudinal analysis of movement observations. Informal data collection from parents, teachers and the head of the school through meetings and email communication are also included. This chapter offers a clear example of the manner of support that the private practitioner can offer to the school. It also offers a gentle introduction for the lay reader to the culture of the school.

School violence is also the theme of Chapter 2, the second contribution from the USA. With teenage violence on the rise, and incidents of shooting making their way into national and international media, the need to intervene early, and ideally in a school environment, appears vital. The violence prevention programme prepared, delivered and evaluated by Lynn Koshland has all the features of a creative adaptation of therapy work (dance movement therapy in this case) into a preventive approach. Through a short-term intervention programme of 12 weeks, Lynn demonstrates the positive outcomes of a reduction in aggressive behaviour and bullying in a primary school. The findings are based on quantitative data collected from the pupils participating in the study, and from the teachers and from observations made by a social work student assisting with the project.

Interestingly, Chapter 3, the last chapter relating to dance movement psychotherapy in mainstream schools (Vicky Karkou, Ailsa Fullarton and Susan Scarth) also deals with prevention (it is framed as a mental health promotion programme). The key features of this work that make it different from the other two chapters are:

1. it involves young adolescents at risk of developing mental health problems in secondary education

2. through a whole school approach, this project targets members of teaching staff as an important first step before engaging young people, who are at risk of developing mental health problems, in a brief dance movement psychotherapy group
3. finally, it is evaluated using both qualitative and quantitative methods within a mixed design that includes a small randomized controlled trial (RCT). Although the sample is too small to draw firm conclusions regarding the effectiveness of the particular intervention with this client group, the study offers an example of practice and ways to evaluate this practice that can be useful for similar work in the future.

Two case studies follow from dramatherapy, both of which make distinctive contributions. Chapter 4, from Jo Christensen, refers to work completed in a learning support unit within a community college for young people aged from 11–19. Jo refers to her work with one boy in particular who was excluded from mainstream school due to aggressive behaviour, subsequently being placed in the learning support centre as a way of attempting to reintegrate him partially into mainstream teaching. Dramatherapy was used as an intervention that supported this transition, as evaluation results indicate. A valuable description of the process of work is also included, illustrating useful interventions as viewed from the boy's own perspective.

The second case study in dramatherapy (Chapter 5), which comes from Sri Lanka, is equally brief and innovative. Its innovative character derives not only from the location of the intervention (there is no tradition of dramatherapy in Sri Lanka) but also from the ways in which solution-focused brief therapy is integrated with dramatherapy theory and practice. Genevieve Smyth from the UK describes her trip to Sri Lanka and how she sets up this work in a school in Colombo for children dealing with high expectations and responsibilities, loss and unresolved conflict. The methods she uses to evaluate her practice remain creative and thus congruent to the creative components of the therapeutic intervention. Examples of her creative collection of information involve session logs, play-based methods of expression (e.g. life maps, social games and group building exercises), reflective discussion and personal process records, alongside open-ended interviews with staff.

The third dramatherapy contribution (Chapter 6) comes from Toby Quibell, in North England, who argues for the value of dramatherapy as an intervention with an impact upon the whole school context and a contribution towards the 'emotional curriculum'. The 136 children involved in this study are seen as disaffected – that is, they present behavioural problems that make it difficult to engage them in the learning process. The chapter concludes that a clearly defined dramatherapy intervention (Toby calls it Action GroupSkills Intervention, AGI), tested in a randomized control environment design, is more effective compared to the control group (a curriculum study group) in terms of reducing disaffection. Furthermore, he provides suggestions that positive effects last for longer. The thorough, quantitative research design and the large sample included in this study add credit to the conclusions reached and provide a clear evidence base for future work.

Shifting to music therapy, Emma Pethybridge and James Robertson (Chapter 7) raise an interesting point: the need to develop new models when working in a setting in which the educational context has a more central role. They term their approach Educational Music Therapy and evaluate its application within brief interventions in schools with children with additional support needs. Video recording has been one of the different types of data collection included in the project, alongside direct observation and checklists completed by parents and teachers. The video recording was made into a DVD which was shown to music specialists and instrumental instructors as a way of encouraging further data collection. Collaborative work between services, and between the music therapists and filmmakers, was at the foundations of this work.

The need to develop a new model of work when situated in a school environment is also acknowledged by Unnur Ottarsdottir in Chapter 8. Given the differences of backgrounds between the author of this chapter and the authors of Chapter 7 (Unnur is an art therapist practising in Iceland, while Emma and James are music therapists based in the UK), the call to develop new ways of working within education becomes even more significant. The particular model suggested by Unnur called Art Educational Therapy, which is an amalgamation of art therapy and educational therapy in which both psychological and learning outcomes are considered. Her model emerged from the use of grounded theory, with five case studies with children with specific learning difficulties associated with stress or trauma and using multiple methods of data collection (e.g. artwork, case notes and coursework, interviews with parents and standardized questionnaires before and after the intervention).

Frances Prokofiev, in Chapter 9, the last of the chapters dealing with work delivered in mainstream schools, highlights the value of image-making within art therapy as a supporting factor in the life of a particular child waiting to be placed with long-term foster parents. Frances follows a retrospective review of the abundance of images created by this child and argues that images offered containment during a period of transition and thus enabled the child to cope with the impermanence of his home situation.

In the second part of the book (Part II), the reader will find different types of interventions dealing primarily with children with autism. Research studies of girls with Rett Syndrome and severe learning difficulties are also included. This section of the book starts with a contribution from Hilda Wengrower (Chapter 10) about dance movement therapy. Hilda's chapter is based on the analysis of reflective notes kept by three of her former students. The notes were taken during the students' placement as part of their training to become dance movement therapists in Barcelona. Hilda concentrates on mirroring, in particular, as a key concept in dance movement therapy and an essential way of working with children with autism or pervasive developmental disorder. She draws parallels with, and clarifies distinctions from, similar concepts found in developmental psychology (e.g. imitation, attunement, kinaesthetic empathy and empathetic reflection). Through thematic analysis of her students' reflective notes, she argues for the need to deepen our understanding of mirroring to take into account the therapist's expectations and anxieties, and to sustain uncertainty or the feeling of not knowing.

Next, in Chapter 11, Lynn Tytherleigh and Vicky Karkou present a case study of a brief dramatherapy group with two children within the autistic spectrum. Relying primarily on Lynn's participant observation as a therapist, and observation of video recordings of sessions, this study identifies significant moments in therapy that indicate relationship building. Both one-to-one and group interactions have emerged with varied character. These interactions are discussed in relation to Sherborne's (2001) developmental movement and Jennings' (1990) model of Embodiment, Projection and Role (EPR). The study shows that although movement work is particularly important, children with autism can engage in role playing, and thus symbolic work, especially when the child's own worldview and preferred themes are used as the topic of their symbolic play.

The role of symbolic work and imagination with children with autism is further discussed in Chapter 12 by art therapist Fuyuko Takeda. Fuyuko presents aspects of her doctoral study in which she used a mixed design to explore this concept further. Although the quantitative components of the study were limited, qualitative findings based on case study material have illustrated that it is possible for children with autism to use their imagination and possibly be supported in this through the use of art therapy.

The series of case studies that focus on the process of the therapeutic work finishes with the case study presented by Jo Tomlinson in music therapy (Chapter 13). Jo, using a hermeneutic phenomenological approach, discusses her work with one child with autism whom she sees for two years, and identifies certain themes that are potentially relevant to working with this client group. For example, she refers to an initial stage during which the child preferred working on his own, followed by the development of interactive play. Specific interventions are discussed as contributing factors in the child's shift from initially engaging with the instruments only to a subsequent musical engagement with the therapist.

The degree to which specific interventions can be particularly useful for enabling communication with children with severe developmental difficulties is also the subject of the single case, multiple probe design (a variant of multiple baseline design) study completed by Cochavit Elefant. In this study (Chapter 14) Cochavit works with seven girls with Rett syndrome, aged 5–10, who are based at a special needs centre in Israel. The aim of the study is to identify intentional choice making, learning abilities, nonconventional communicative behaviours and song preferences. The quantitative findings of the study make suggestions for the role of pre-composed children's songs in music therapy in terms of providing motivation, enabling learning and demonstrating preferences. Qualitative findings highlight that children's emotional responses and different expressions can be seen as communicative acts with meaning, and thus of value, when communication with the primary carers is concerned.

The last contribution (Chapter 15) comes from Australia. Music therapist Katrina McFerran and special educator Jennifer Stephenson joined forces to study the benefits of music therapy, in school settings, for children with severe disabilities. Following a quantitative methodology they explore the extent to which music therapy interventions can play an important role in producing more communicative acts amongst students with severe learning disabilities. They compare this with interaction between the students and the same therapist during other activities that include neither music nor singing. The study used an ABAB design that involved video recording of non-music sessions (A) alternating with music sessions (B), and indicated that there was a small advantage for music sessions in terms of student responsiveness and vocalizations. However, the authors also suggest that the interaction between the therapist and the student was in itself probably more important than the type of activity. They also conclude that the study highlighted design limitations, and argue for the need to develop more refined coding schemes and more individualized analysis of the behaviour of the participating students.

The same contribution from Katrina and Jennifer also includes a useful discussion of evidence-based practice, and suggests that there are certain aspects of arts therapies work that can be quantified and rigorously studied. This, along with discussion in other parts of the book on qualitative approaches to arts therapies practice, offers the reader a wide range of possibilities that reflect a similarly wide range of therapeutic interventions and research interests.

The concluding section provides various suggestions for further research in terms of the theory, research and practice of arts therapies in schools.

REFERENCES

Bunt, L. (1994) *Music Therapy: An Art Beyond Words.* London and New York: Routledge.

Bush, J. (1997) *The Handbook of School Art Therapy.* Springfield, IL: Charles C. Thomas.

Cochrane Collaboration (2009) Cochrane Collaboration – contact details of methods, groups and fields. Avaialble at www.cochrane.org/contact/mwgfield.htm#38, accessed on 13 May 2009.

Coe, R. (1999) 'A manifesto for evidence-based education.' Available at www.cemcentre.org/renderpage.asp?linkID=30317000, accessed on 13 May 2009.

Crimmens, P. (2006) *Drama Therapy and Storymaking in Special Education.* London: Jessica Kingsley Publishers.

Davies, P. (1999) 'What is evidence-based education?' *British Journal of Educational Studies 47,* 2, 108–121.

Eccles, M., Freemantle, N. and Mason, J. (2001) 'Using Systematic Reviews in Clinical Guideline Development.' In M. Egger, G.D. Smith and D.G. Atman (eds) *Systematic Reviews in Health Care: Meta-analysis in Context.* London: British Medical Journal Books, 400–418.

Evans, K. and Dubowski, J. (2001) *Art Therapy and Children on the Autistic Spectrum: Beyond Words.* London: Jessica Kingsley Publishers.

Fonagy, P., Target, M., Cottrell, D., Philips, J. and Kurtz, Z. (2002) *What Works for Whom? A Critical Review of Treatments for Children and Adolescents.* New York: Guilford Press.

Gilroy, A. (2006) *Art Therapy, Research and Evidence-based Practice.* London: Sage.

Hargreaves, D. (1997) 'In defense of research for evidence-based teaching: a rejoinder to Martyn Hammersley.' *British Educational Research Journal 23,* 405–419.

Heal, M. and Wigram, T. (1993) *Music Therapy in Health and Education.* London: Jessica Kingsley Publishers.

Jennings, S. (1987) 'Introduction.' In S. Jennings (ed.) *Dramatherapy: Theory and Practice 1.* London: Routledge, xv–xx.

Jennings, S. (1990) *Dramatherapy with Families, Groups and Individuals. Waiting in the Wings.* London: Jessica Kingsley Publishers.

Jennings, S. (1995) (ed.) *Dramatherapy with Children and Adolescents.* London: Routledge.

Karkou, V. (1998) 'A descriptive evaluation of the practice of arts therapies in the UK.' Unpublished PhD thesis. School of Education, University of Manchester.

Karkou, V. (1999) 'Art therapy in education: findings from a nation-wide survey in arts therapies.' *Inscape: The Journal of the BAAT 4*, 2, 62–70.

Karkou, V. and Glasman, J. (2004) 'Arts, education and society: the role of the arts in promoting the emotional well-being and social inclusion of young people.' *Support for Learning 19*, 2, 56–64.

Karkou, V. and Sanderson, P. (2000) 'Dance movement therapy in UK education.' *Research in Dance Education 1*, 1, 69–85.

Karkou, V. and Sanderson, P. (2001) 'Dance movement therapy in the UK: current orientations of a field emerging from dance education.' *European P.E. Review 7*, 2, 137–155.

Karkou, V. and Sanderson, P. (2006) *Arts Therapies: A Research-based Map of the Field.* Edinburgh: Elsevier.

Laban, R. (1960) *The Mastery of Movement.* London: MacDonald and Evans.

Martinsone, K., Karkou, V. and Nazarova, N. (2009) 'Comparison of the organisation of art therapy practice in Latvia, in the UK and in Russia.' *Collection of Scientific Papers 2009.* Riga: Riga Stradins University.

McFarlane, P. (2005) *Dramatherapy: Raising Children's Self-esteem and Developing Emotional Stability.* London: David Fulton Publishers.

McNiff, S. (1998) *Art-Based Research.* London: Jessica Kingsley Publishers.

Moriya, D. (2000) *Art Therapy in Schools: Effective Integration of Art Therapists in Schools.* Israel: Turbo.

Payne, H. (1992) 'Introduction.' In H. Payne (ed.) *Dance Movement Therapy: Theory and Practice.* London and New York: Tavistock/Routledge, 1–17.

Peter, M. (1998) '"Good for them, or what?" The arts and pupils with SEN.' *British Journal of Special Education 25*, 4, 168–172.

Sanderson, P. (1996) 'Dance within the national P.E. curriculum of England and Wales.' *The European Physical Education Review 2*, 1, 54–63.

Sherborne, V. (2001) *Developmental Movement for Children.* London: Worth Publishing.

Stein-Safran, D. (2002) *Art Therapy and ADHD: Diagnostic and Therapeutic Approaches.* London: Jessica Kingsley Publishers.

Valente, L. and Fontana, D. (1991) 'Dramatherapy and Psychological Change.' In G.D. Wilson (ed.) *Psychology and Performing Arts.* Amsterdam and Zeilinger: Swets, 121–131.

Wadsworth-Hervey, L. (2000) *Artistic Inquiry in Dance/Movement Therapy: Creative Alternatives for Research.* Springfield, IL: Charles C. Thomas.

Wengrower, H. (2001) 'Arts therapies in educational settings: An intercultural encounter.' *The Arts in Psychotherapy 28*, 2, 109–115.

Wigram, T. (1993) 'Music Therapy Research to Meet the Demands of Health and Educational Services.' In M. Heal and T. Wigram (eds) *Music Therapy in Health and Education.* London: Jessica Kingsley Publishers.

Waller, D. (1992) 'Different things to different people: art therapy in Britain – a brief survey of its history and current development.' *The Arts in Psychotherapy 19*, 87–92.

Warwick, A. (1995) 'Music Therapy in the Education Service: Research with Autistic Children and their Mothers.' In T. Wigram, B. Saperston and R. West (eds) *The Art and Science of Music Therapy: A Handbook.* Switzerland: Harwood Academic Publications, 209–225.

Part I

Mainstream Schools

Chapter 1

From the Dance Studio to the Classroom

Translating the Clinical Dance Movement Psychotherapy Experience into a School Context

Suzi Tortora

INTRODUCTION

Setting the scene

> The bubble bee was such a bully; even when asked she would not stop stinging everyone. One day she went far away. When she came back everyone was so surprised that she was better. She listened and was friendly and best of all she wasn't stinging anyone. Everyone wanted to know what had happened. She said she met someone that helped her feel better and now she could be nice... (Salina 2007. DMP client, seven years old.)

The excerpt above is from a story written, directed and performed by Salina,[2] aged seven, during one of her weekly private dance movement psychotherapy sessions. It was developed from the activity called ' complete the story' (Crenshaw 2004), which invites the child to add her own ending to a story that involves some type of conflict representative of her own internal issues. The core of the story depicts an initially out-of-control animal who one day disappears. When she returns, she has

2 The names in this case study have been changed to protect confidentiality.

changed. The child is asked to decide what happened to the animal upon leaving her community, and what she explains to her friends upon her return. In Salina's version of the story the bubble bee tells her family and friends that she finds a wise person to share her concerns with. Through this person, she is taught how to share her feelings more appropriately, is able to return home, and is welcomed and successfully integrated into her community. This story was written a year and a half into Salina's private dance movement psychotherapy sessions. In its sincerity and simplicity it depicts how she experienced the effects of her sessions.

Salina was referred to dance movement psychotherapy because of concerns her parents and the school had about her extremely disruptive, volatile, emotional and physical behaviour. In school these behaviours manifested through controlling and bullying actions. Salina was unable to calm herself down when upset, and had unpredictable, sudden outbursts that suggested difficulties with emotional and physical regulation. This case study explores how the use of dance, body awareness and relaxation techniques, story writing and dance-play activities, along with music, were used to assist Salina in learning how to gain control over her difficult behaviours.

LITERATURE REVIEW

Over the past 60 years, the expressive and healing aspects of dance have been widely explored as a method for psychological change (Bernstein 1981; Halprin 2004; Levy 2005; Tortora 2006). Through both group and individual dance movement psychotherapy sessions, participants gain awareness of feelings, thoughts and experiences that may be felt but not easily expressed. It is in the body that these experiences are held. Since movement is the initial and primary language of the body, movement-based activities create metaphoric entry into the emotional/feeling self (Halprin 2004; Tortora 2006). By moving these feelings, using the tools of improvisational dance, music and theatrical explorations, psychodynamic structures that underlie the mover's perspective and way of being in the world are revealed, explored and developed. The aim is to facilitate improved functioning on all levels of an individual's life.

The field of dance education has also used the tools of dance and dance making to support personal growth. Dance scholars have widely researched the effectiveness of school-based dance programmes to enhance the academic learning process (Gilbert 2006; Laban 1968; Stinson 2004.

Dance educational programmes have been offered within the actual classroom curriculum to provide experiential learning of all academic subjects, often providing a bridge between subjects, creating cross-modal learning opportunities. Dance movement psychotherapy sessions conducted in school settings are typically offered for children with special needs such as autism, attention deficit disorders, hyperactivity, communication difficulties, conduct disorders and issues with relating, in order to support improved socialization, self-expression, attention, academic learning, body awareness and body control (Levy 2005; Tortora 2001; see also Wengrower in Chapter 10 of this book). Dance movement psychotherapy has also successfully been implemented in bullying, peace, and violence prevention school programmes (Beardall 1996, 2005; Beardall, Bergman and Surrey 2007; Kornblum 2002; Koshland and Wittaker 2004).

In this chapter a model of intervention will be discussed that uses the psychodynamic elements revealed in a private dance movement psychotherapy treatment to improve classroom functioning (Tortora 2006). This model, called 'Ways of Seeing', highlights the role of the clinical psychotherapeutic setting as a liaison between the home and school environment.

THE STUDY

Research questions

This case study systematically explores how the 'Ways of Seeing' model has supported change in Salina's school experience. The following questions guided this inquiry:

1. Can the metaphoric process of dance expression, as revealed in the dance movement psychotherapy sessions, support a child's improvement in the school setting?
2. Can physical stress and affect regulation methods used in the dance movement psychotherapy setting be translated into behavioural improvement for an elementary school-age child?

The Ways of Seeing programme

'Ways of Seeing' is a comprehensive theoretical, clinical and research-based programme that was developed over a 20-year period. It is based on an extensive variety of sources, including the nonverbal observational principles of Laban Movement Analysis (LMA); the discipline of authentic movement (Adler 2002); dance movement psychotherapy practice; and early childhood developmental principles (Tortora 2006). Underlying all components of the programme is the essential goal of supporting social and emotional expression, stabilization and mental health. This is done within the context of developing a secure relationship between the therapist, the child and the family by providing a safe therapeutic 'holding' environment (Winnicott 1965), from which the patients feel comfortable enough to share their concerns.

A key element of the 'Ways of Seeing' programme, which has played a significant role in this case study, is analysing how the child's nonverbal movement style reveals information about how the child regulates herself on an emotional and physiological level. This interplay between emotional and physical/sensory regulation can significantly influence how the child experiences and expresses herself, and how she behaves in the surroundings – which, in turn, influences how she forms relationships with others.

One of the most important aspects of dance movement psychotherapy practice that was instituted in this study was 'starting where the patient is at' (Bernstein 1981; Levy 2005; Tortora 2006). This classic phrase enables the therapist to attune to the patient, letting the patient's own particular needs and nonverbal style direct and guide the session. Following the child's lead, rather than imposing preconceived ideas about how the therapeutic intervention should unfold, immediately enables the child to feel respected and listened to.

The activities of each session were organized with the four dynamic processes of the Ways of Seeing programme in mind (Tortora 2006). These activities may occur either simultaneously or as separate elements supporting the developing relationship and the unfolding metaphoric content of the activities. These dynamic processes are as follows.

1. *Establishing rapport*: all activities aim to enhance the social/emotional and communicative development of the child. This is a key element of dance movement psychotherapy practice that differentiates our work from other body-oriented approaches such as occupational, physical and somatic movement-based therapy. These methods focus on movement rehabilitation and re-education. Dance movement therapists are trained to provide psychological support using movement, dance and the body as added tools for

expression and intervention. I emphasize this point by calling the practice 'dance movement psychotherapy'.

2. *Expressing feelings*: the establishment of this relationship enables the child to become comfortable exploring deeper feelings, emotions and traumatic events. All activities are designed to support the child for such exploration, often revealing experiences the child may or may not be conscious of from his or her past or present experience.
3. *Building skills*: the movement and body-based nature of the activities of the session also provides the opportunity to build physical, cognitive and communicative skills within the context of the psychological and physiological themes that arise.
4. *Healing dance*: dance, movement and dance-play activities can have an intrinsically joyful and healing element to them. Dance-play activities (Tortora 2006) include the movement, dance, play and story-telling elements that develop during a session. Dance identifies the embodied, improvisational and choreographed nature of the activities; play references the creative, playful and pretend aspects of the activities that unfold.

Borrowing the concept from dance education, the actual structure of the sessions is a dance class format providing external form and organization (Gilbert 2006: Stinson 2004). A therapeutic focus dominates the content of this dance class format:

1. *Warm-up*: this includes verbal processing of how the past week at home and school went; sensory–body regulating activities; and a Chace dance therapy circle activity, in which each person takes turns leading a movement/dance action that involves moving different parts of the body in response to music (Bernstein 1981; Chaiklin 1975; Levy 2005).
2. *Improvisational exploration of a story theme or movement concept conceived during the warm-up*: this is child-directed, taking the form of partner dance explorations or elaborate, enacted story-telling dance-plays. Through the story, the nature of the child's difficulties is expressed, explored and processed. Other family members are actively involved in this section of the session. Including family members in embodied play scenarios enables the underlying family

dynamics to unfold and be explored through this process (Harvey 1990, 1994).

3. *Cool-down/centring activity*: this begins ten minutes before the end of the 60-minute session to create a transition from active expression of emotional themes to containment, emotional and physical regulation, organization, and closure of the session.

Attachment issues were also considered during this treatment (Ainsworth 1978; Main and Hesse 1990). They were addressed through the lens of affective and physiological regulatory methods. Emotional and physiological regulation involves the ability to process emotional and sensory information from the body and the environment in an organized way (Greenspan and Glovinsky 2007; Williamson and Anzalone 2001). Interventions include identifying emotional and physical behaviours that reveal 'dysregulation'; assessing the role of the current environment that may be contributing to them; and implementing specific physical methods designed to improve organization by controlling sensory input to activate more functional brain mechanisms. Techniques involving body and breath awareness, relaxation and internal body co-ordination activities, using concepts from Bartenieff fundamentals (a series of dynamic movement sequences that support internal body co-ordination, balance, integrity and core support; Bartenieff and Lewis 1980); and Body–Mind Centering® (a method of movement analysis and re-education developed by Bonnie Bainbridge Cohen, based on foundational body systems that include developmental movement, reflexes and basic neurological patterns; Cohen 1997), created experiential ways to explore regulation. Weaving these activities into the dance-play stories enabled Salina and her mum to explore issues of their relationship, which had manifested in emotional dysregulation.

Methodology

Data collection occurred over a two-year period using the 'Ways of Seeing' daily note form, behavioural descriptions worksheet and movement signature impressions (Tortora 2006). The *daily note form* chronicled the activities of each session as it unfolded. Specific events that occurred during a session were analysed in more detail using the behavioural descriptions worksheet. Longitudinal analysis of Salina's nonverbal behaviours was conducted using the movement signature impressions. Movement Signature

Impressions (MSI) is a nonverbal observational tool I developed, to guide the practitioner's observations about the individual's nonverbal personal and interactional movement style.

Included in each of these forms is a self-observation section that tracks the therapist's reflective experiences and [countertransference] reactions (Tortora 2006). There are three elements to this self-observation method: witnessing, kinaesthetic seeing and kinaesthetic empathy. *Witnessing* (W) is adapted from authentic movement practice. It provides a detailed description of the child's actions, and tracks the therapist's first thoughts and reactions regarding the child's actions. *Kinaesthetic seeing* (KS) tracks the therapist's sensorial reactions during the session. *Kinaesthetic empathy* (KE) tracks the therapist's emotional reactions during the session. An example of how these are incorporated within the main data collection forms can be found in the behavioural descriptions worksheet presented in Figure 1.1.

Additional data were collected through email correspondence and individual sessions with both parents, and through school reports, as well as monthly phone meetings with the school principal, special education teacher and classroom teacher. Following qualitative research practice (Bogdan and Biklen 1998; Erickson and Mohatt 1982; Janesick 1994; Merriam 1998), analysing a variety of methods of documentation provided a rich array of sources to examine the effects of the dance movement psychotherapy approach on the child's school performance.

Findings and discussion

PRESENTATION OF SALINA

Salina began dance movement psychotherapy treatment at age six years eight months during her first grade year in primary school. Both parents had been concerned about her difficult behaviour, which included out-of-control, volatile physical and verbal outbursts that occurred unpredictably; disrespect for authority figures; and difficulty with limit setting, especially when told 'no', coupled with an underlying issue of low self-esteem and overall emotional fragility that appeared to be masked by a tough, bullying persona. Concerns about her behaviour were also surfacing in her first grade classroom, as evidenced in her teacher's semester report, under the categories 'areas needing improvement' and 'areas of significant concern':

> Salina sometimes becomes irritated when she is told 'no' and acts out inappropriately with verbal remarks...she is sometimes discouraged and loses focus when an activity is challenging for her. Salina is

Behavioural descriptions worksheet

Name of child: Salina

Date: 12/16/05

Age: 6.8 years

Date of birth: 4/4/1999

Observer: Suzi

Detailed general description	Possible influences: internal/ environmental	What does it communicate to you?	Detailed description of body movements	'Try on' action: describe feelings/ insights	Movement-based interventions
– Initially won't get out of car, mum enters room very apologetic – takes responsibility, S upset with her for she forgot to bring dance clothes. – S comes to door, flinging body at mother, screaming, swinging arms at mum hitting/ slapping, mum tries to grab her arms and S pulls away quickly but comes back with more swings, S will not look at me –	– Internal: extreme anxiety about new place; defensive about coming to therapy; fright/ flight response, 'neuroceptive' lack of safety wondering if any sensory sensitivities/seeking – proprioceptive seeking, consider tactile issues? – External – wondering about the nature of the parent–child relationship; does the mother set limits?	W – wow! She is strong willed, I am concerned that she is so out of control she may run out into the parking lot when a care is coming. Her body is turning red and she seems not to be able to 'turn off' or slow down her actions. I wonder how often this happens; the mum seems at a loss but also not surprised by this behaviour. KS – I feel very alert in my whole body. I will not lose focus	Mum – body – direct eye contact, use of whole body, some are gesturing on occasion; clear body boundaries, sense of containment. Effort – weight and space – light direct use of arms when gesturing; full body weighted sense. Space – near and mid-reach space with arm gestures; full body posturing mostly in place, not much use of space.	So much sadness, pain, fear, despair in both – makes me wonder more about merging kinespheric space, is this demonstrative of S's attempt to actually connect to mum – symbotic senses of self and other, despite the negative results this causes?	Did – stayed calm, consistent, gentle, through even phrasing rhythm (with NV actions as well as vocal tone) – no surprises or sudden changes. Gestural actions with clear efforts using flow and space – direct/indirect Shaping – fluctuating between vertical centred stance and full body shaping around my legs, with softness.

Behavioural descriptions worksheet *cont.*

Name of child: Salina | Date: 12/16/05

Age: 6.8 years | Date of birth: 4/4/1999 | Observer: Suzi

Detailed general description	Possible influences: internal/ environmental	What does it communicate to you?	Detailed description of body movements	'Try on' action: describe feelings/ insights	Movement-based interventions
says she wants to go home – won't come in, runs back out door, into parking lot, locks self in car. – Mum seems distraught, at a loss about what to do. – I speak to her and say it may take time. – S's behaviors take up the whole session.		for one moment, the situation feels so unpredictable. KE – my heart goes out to mum, who seems so distraught, underneath her efforts to hold it together – I feel deep anguish as I observe her. As I observe S, I sense extreme fear and such a sense of being out of control. I yearn for some protection, but not sure if S feels this. If she does it might be unconscious.	Shape – concave torso. S – efforts – time, space, weight: fast, indirect, heavy. Phrasing – explosive, impactive, erratic full body actions as she throws her body. Body – mostly full body actions. Space – merging kinespheric space as throws body on mum and car door, large use of space scattered pathways.		Try – maintain this sense of presence – this behaviour may occur for a few sessions to come! Attempt to establish eye contact with S even if it is fleeting – be reassuring. Look for moments of calm emotionally and/or physically and mirror them. Look for positive moments of interaction between mum and S and praise them. Create a safe space following her cues.

Figure 1.1: Behavioural descriptions worksheet. See p.33 for definitions of W, KS and KE.

> working on maintaining her friendships and regulating control of her social/emotional behaviour...[she] has a need for dominance in social situations. I sincerely believe Salina is a kind and generous girl who needs practice demonstrating these innate attributes... Her distractibility has been an issue...as it is disruptive to the class, and she has not been able to use strategies to settle herself. (First grade teacher, semester report 2005, prior to Salina beginning DMP.)

The school recommended that the parents seek therapeutic intervention. Salina's parents thought a creative arts therapeutic approach would best suit their daughter's needs, supporting her highly creative and energetic theatrical strengths.

WORKING WITH SALINA IN DANCE MOVEMENT PSYCHOTHERAPY

Salina's difficult behaviour was immediately apparent during the initial session, when mum could not get her to leave the car. When she eventually came in, she flung her whole body at her mother in a weighted manner, slapping her mother, screaming at her, grabbing her arm and attempting to drag her out of the room. Mum was distressed but tried to stay calm and neutral. These behaviours instantly brought to question Salina's level of anxiety, sense of safety, and difficulties with internal regulation; along with a need to learn more about the nature of the parent–child relationship. The behavioural descriptions worksheet notes for that session describe my immediate impressions.

What does it communicate to you?

> *Witnessing*: Salina is strong-willed, I am concerned that she is so out of control she may run into the parking lot when a car is coming. Her body is turning red and she seems not to be able to 'turn off' or slow down her actions. I wonder how often this happens mum seems at a loss but also not surprised by this behaviour.
>
> *Kinaesthetic seeing*: I feel very alert in my whole body. I will not lose focus for one moment, the situation feels so unpredictable.
>
> *Kinaesthetic empathy*: my heart goes out to this mum who seems so distraught, underneath her efforts to hold it together – I feel deep anguish as I observe her. As I observe Salina, I sense extreme fear and such a sense of being out of control. I yearn for some protection, but not sure if Salina feels this. (If she does it, it might be unconscious.)

> *Movement interventions*: try – maintain a sense of presence – this behaviour may occur for several sessions to come. Attempt to establish eye contact with Salina even if it is fleeting – be reassuring. Look for moments of calm emotionally and/or physically and mirror them. Look for positive moments of interaction between mum and Salina and praise them. Create a safe space, by following her cues.

A safe space with clear boundaries was created by limiting extra stimulation, being calm and direct and avoiding getting overexcited by Salina's out-of-control behaviours, while staying firm about what behaviours were acceptable and which were not. No hitting or hurting any of us, including herself, was a paramount rule. Setting this boundary provided a much needed protective container for Salina. It explicated that the adults would help her when she could not maintain control of herself. Structuring sessions in a dance class format enabled the opening warm-up, using very soothing music, to become a time to slow Salina's body down through breath awareness and massage. It was a time for Salina and mum to talk calmly about the events of the week.

Initially it was difficult for Salina to remain quiet in body and mind, often jumping up to stop her mum from revealing something that caused her anguish. Over time she was able to maintain this relaxed state, which eventually extended for 20 to 30 minutes of the hour-long session.

An active sharing of movement ideas in a Chace format followed. This included taking turns sharing, trying on and developing different movement ideas we each contributed. At times Salina allowed the calm music to continue to play, at other times she chose a song from current teen pop culture. Salina demonstrated a terrific sense of rhythm and flow throughout her body. However, the phrasing of her actions was punctuated by explosive, accented gestures and full body actions, during which she would wildly 'throw' her body parts as if to scatter them with a 'heavy', weighted quality. This was especially apparent when swing dancing with mum. During this favourite activity she would increasingly become more out of control, increasing her tempo and throwing herself at her mother, who tried to enjoy it but verbalized concerns about pain in her back and arms due to the thrust in Salina's actions.

Regulating her physical actions by attuning to her dancing partner through specific dance techniques became the focus of sessions. These included greater awareness of shifting and sharing her body weight with her partner; maintaining her weight over her feet with full body alignment; working with maintaining an established tempo; and increased control of her gestures and actions, using strength and lightness. Turn-taking activities improved her social awareness of self and others. All sessions concluded with a centring activity involving breathing and lengthening up the spine while matching the quality of a melodic chime bar instrument that gradually decreased in tone. A moment of silent, calm breathing completed the session. These explorations, repeated each session, created new, deeply felt body experiences in a safe (holding) environment with mum.

In concert with these activities in sessions were monthly school phone meetings in which the therapist described the metaphoric importance of Salina's efforts to gain physical control and internal regulation. Analogies were made between Salina's lack of body boundaries and thrusting physical behaviour in sessions, and her abrupt, intense manner in the classroom. Her second grade teacher's specific concerns were: not waiting her turn to provide answers, inserting herself into conversations, pushing and shoving in a queue, physically taking up extra space by looking at children's work during test taking, and being 'desperate to have a partner, but when she gets one she is too dominant' (discussion with teacher, 2006). During these phone sessions we discussed ways to translate the dance-play activities into classroom strategies. The teachers learned to recognize when Salina's behaviours were caused by too much sensory or emotional input, revealing her inability to regulate/modulate herself, rather than a wilful acting out.

By the end of this school year, the teacher described Salina as still being bossy, however, she was becoming a '...magnetic leader. Children gravitate toward her, but still do get irritated with her'. She described Salina as '...the Queen Bee. She is wonderful and powerful!' (Discussion with teacher, 2007.) In sessions we focused on honing this power so that it did not push others away. The improvisational story theme evolved into dance-plays about a queen (Salina) who would trick her subjects (mum and the therapist), appearing nice at the beginning of the dance ball, but then deceiving them by stealing their clothes while they danced. Our emotional pain about the loss of the nice queen, and what her motivations were, were discussed extensively. Over time, we and the queen became sisters, gallivanting both separately and together in the woods, presenting each other with gifts. At times someone would appear lost, and we would work together to find her. Gaiety abounded as we enjoyed each other's company, marvelled over our lovely dresses, and shared dancing moves.

As Salina's behaviour continued to improve at school, Salina began to talk about other children who might benefit from the work we were doing. These discussions enabled Salina to neutralize her difficulties, viewing them as issues other children also experience. During monthly phone calls we discussed ways that Salina could be recognized for her increased ability to stay emotionally and physically regulated at school. We spoke of activities and concepts we did in session that might help the whole classroom. I provided numerous classroom activity suggestions incorporating concepts from our sessions that could benefit all the students.

CONCLUSIONS

This case study demonstrates how the expressive and healing aspects of an individual dance movement psychotherapy treatment were translated into the school setting to support a young child's improvement. Specific to this method is that the metaphoric implications of the dance and body awareness activities implemented in the clinical setting provided increased insight for the school staff to best support Salina. In the words of the school principal:

> Dr Tortora [also] helped us to see the reasons behind why the student was acting in these ways. By learning about the emotional piece behind the behaviour, I believe we are more able to be compassionate with this student and her family. By knowing why she is doing something, we are better able to communicate with her and help her learn more appropriate coping techniques. (School principal, 2007.)

The emotional symbolism of Salina's behaviours was revealed through examination of her actions. Nonverbal movement analysis revealed explosive and accelerated movement phrases punctuated by accented gestures and full-body actions using heavy, passive body weight. Salina appeared to be throwing her limbs and body around, disconnecting her body parts from her whole. These actions 'scattered' her emotionally and physically, contributing to her already fragile affective and physiological/sensorial systems. On a relational level, as Salina pulled, dragged and hit her mum, she sent a complex nonverbal message, seeming to lose her independent sense of self in an attempt to merge with mum, while at the same time resisting mum through the abrupt, aggressive quality of her actions. In school these actions translated to difficulty in forming peer relationships, extreme bossiness verging on bullying, impulse control issues and overall disrespect toward the teacher and students. As described by the principal, Salina demonstrated 'difficulty with boundaries, needing to control situations, and defiance'.

Analysis of these behaviours within the context of the 'Ways of Seeing' sense of body concept correlated Salina's bodily felt experience with her observable actions and behaviours related to affect, mood and physiological dysregulation. The mind–body–emotional link associated with the sense of body concept revealed that this scattered and weighted, nonverbal movement style expressed a lack of internal integration, creating a sense of body self that greatly contributed to Salina's emotional, labile, fearful and controlling behaviours. On a deeply felt, experiential and metaphoric body level, Salina did not feel integrated. This lack of internal and physical integration made it very difficult to feel individuated within external relationships, causing her to strive to control her interactions with others.

The dance movement psychotherapy treatment provided an avenue to enable Salina to develop a sense of individuation between self and other, with activities that literally helped her feel her body moving with integrity and fluidity. She learned to 'hold her own weight' as she partner danced while healing her emotional attachment with mum. As mum learned how to set limits with her daughter, she established her parental role, creating a safer environment. Through body awareness and relaxation activities Salina experienced how to become aware of when her body was dysregulated. This opened up discussions about how this dysregulation manifested behaviourally, enabling her to make a cognitive link between her emotional and physical behaviour.

This information was discussed with the classroom teachers to help them identify when the school environment was contributing to her regulatory difficulties. Creating classroom activities that Salina could participate in with the class enabled her to demonstrate her improved control, and normalized her experience.

At the time of writing, Salina's dance movement psychotherapy sessions still continue, with the focus on creating more experiences that will help Salina improve her ability to identify and regulate her stress and mood dysregulation. Her school principal summarized our efforts and goals:

> Over the two years, we have seen amazing improvement in this student's behaviour and in her ability to relate to others. Of course, it is still a work in progress. I believe that this amazing progress is due partially to the wisdom and insight of Dr Suzi Tortora, coupled with our team approach, so the student is receiving consistent messages from all of the adults around her. (School principal, written summary report 2007.)

REFERENCES

Adler, J. (2002) *Offering from the Conscious Body: The Discipline of Authentic Movement.* Rochester, VT: Inner Traditions.

Ainsworth, M.D.S. (1978) *Patterns of Attachment: a Psychological Study of the Strange Situation.* Hillsdale, NJ: Erlbaum.

Bartenieff, I. and Lewis, D. (1980) *Body Movement: Coping with the Environment.* New York: Gordon and Breach Science Publishers, Inc.

Beardall, N. (1996) *Creating a Peaceable School: Confronting Intolerance and Bullying.* Newton, MA: Newton Public Schools.

Beardall, N. (2005) 'Dance the Dream.' In M.C. Powell and V. Marcow Speiser (eds) *The Arts, Education, and Social Change: Little Signs of Hope.* New York: Peter Lang.

Beardall, N., Bergman, S. and Surrey, J. (2007) *Making Connections: Building Community and Gender Dialogue in Secondary Schools.* Cambridge, MA: Educators for Social Responsibility.

Bernstein, P. (1981) *Theory and Methods in Dance-Movement Therapy.* Dubuque, IA: Kendall/Hunt Publishing Company.

Bogdan, R. and Biklen, S.K. (1998) *Qualitative Research for Education: An Introduction to Theory and Methods.* Third edition. Boston, MA: Allyn & Bacon.

Chaiklin, H. (ed.) (1975) *Marion Chase: Her Papers.* Columbia, MD: American Dance Therapy Association.

Cohen, B.B. (1997) *Sensing, Feeling, and Action: the Experiential Anatomy of Body–Mind Centering.* Northampton, MA: Contact Editions.

Crenshaw, D.A. (2004) *Engaging Resistant Children in Therapy.* Rhinebeck, NY: Rhinebeck Child and Family Center Publications.

Erickson, F. and Mohatt, G. (1982) 'Cultural Organization of Participation in Two Classrooms of Indian Students.' In G. Spindler (ed.) *Doing the Ethnography of Schooling: Educational Anthropology in Action.* New York: Holt, Rinehart & Wilson, 134–171.

Gilbert, A.G. (2006) *Brain-compatible Dance Education.* Reston, VA: National Dance Association, American Alliance for Health, Physical Education, Recreation and Dance.

Greenspan, S.I. and Glovinsky, I. (2007) *Children and Babies with Mood Swings: New Insights for Parents and Professionals.* Bethesda, MD: Interdisciplinary Council on Developmental and Learning Disorders.

Halprin, D. (2004) *The Expressive Body in Life, Art and Therapy: Working with Movement, Metaphor and Meaning.* Philadelphia, PA: Jessica Kingsley Publishers.

Harvey, S. (1990) 'Creating a family: an integrated expressive arts approach to the family therapy of young children.' *The Arts in Psychotherapy 18,* 213–222.

Harvey, S. (1994) 'Dynamic play therapy: an integrated expressive arts approach to the family treatment of infants and toddlers.' *Zero to Three 15,* 1, 11–17. August/September.

Janesick, V. (1994) 'The Dance of Qualitative Research Design: Metaphor, Methodolatry, and Meaning.' In N.L. Denzin and Y.S. Lincoln (eds) *Handbook of Qualitative Research,* Thousand Oaks, CA: Sage Publications, 209–219 .

Kornblum, R. (2002) *Disarming the Playground: Violence Prevention through Movement and Pro-social Skills. Training Manual.* Oklahoma City, OK: Wood and Barnes Publishing.

Koshland, L. and Wittaker, J.W.B. (2004) 'Peace through dance/movement: evaluating a violence prevention programme.' *American Journal of Dance Therapy 26,* 2, 69–90.

Laban, R. (1968) *Modern Educational Dance.* (2nd edition, revised L. Ulmann.) London: MacDonald and Evans, Ltd.

Levy, F. J. (2005) *Dance Movement Therapy: a Healing Art.* (Revised edition.) Reston, VA: American Alliance for Health, Physical Education, Recreation and Dance.

Main, M. and Hesse, E. (1990) 'Parents' Unresolved Traumatic Experiences are Related To Infant Disorganized Attachment Status: Is Frightened and/or Frightening Parental Behaviour the Linking Mechanism?' In M. Greenberg, D. Cicchetti and E.M. Cummings (eds) *Attachment in the Preschool Years: Theory, Research and Interventio*n. Chicago, IL: University of Chicago Press, 161–182

Merriam, S. (1998) 'Conducting Effective Interviews.' In S. Merriam *Case Study Research in Education: a Qualitative Approach.* New York: Jossy-Boss.

Stinson, S.W. (2004) 'My Body/Myself: Lessons from Dance Education.' In L. Bresler (ed.) *Knowing Bodies, Feeling Minds: Embodied Knowledge in Arts Education and Schooling.* Dordrecht, The Netherlands: Kluwer, 153–168.

Tortora, S. (2001) 'The use of the "Ways of Seeing" programme with a young child with Rett Syndrome' (doctoral dissertation, Teachers College, Columbia University, 2001). UMI Dissertation Services, 3014818.

Tortora, S. (2006) *The Dancing Dialogue: Using the Communicative Power of Dance with Young Children.* Baltimore, MD: Paul H. Brookes Publishing Co.

Williamson, G.G. and Anzalone, M. (2001) *Sensory Integration and Self-regulation in Infants and Toddlers: Helping very Young Children Interact with their Environment.* Washington, DC: Zero to Three.

Winnicott, D.W. (1965) *The Maturational Processes and the Facilitating Environment.* New York: International Universities Press.

Chapter 2

PEACE through Dance Movement Therapy

The Development and Evaluation of a Violence Prevention Programme in an Elementary School

Lynn Koshland

INTRODUCTION

Setting the scene

School violence and 'peer cruelty' in the forms of bullying, shootings and peer aggression have impacted all parts of the USA and the world, bringing the issue of violence to the forefront of educational concerns (Fried and Fried 2003; Olweus 1993). For example, in the northern part of Norway during the fall of 1982, school-related bullying problems were brought to the media and public attention through the suicidal deaths of three students as a most likely consequence of severe bullying by peers (Olweus 1993). As a result of these tragic events, the Norwegian Ministry of Education implemented a nationwide campaign against bully/victim problems. In recent decades, the USA has been marked by tragic reports of peer abuse and related violence.

Dance movement therapist Fried and her daughter, a clinical psychologist, explored the short-term and long-lasting psychological and emotional scars that bullying can cause and offered a few possible answers to these questions about school violence in their books (Fried and Fried 1996, 2003). They proposed that children involved in school violence might have been victims of abuse themselves, or have displayed continuous problematic behaviours related to difficulties containing and expressing anger that were left untreated. In addition, they stated that the common factor running through the complex problem of school violence is the limited abilities of youth to deal with relationship conflicts (Koshland and Whittaker 2004).

Bullying is defined by Olweus (1993) as inflicting negative aggressive acts repeatedly over time on one or more students. Bullying problems in the schools, if not handled, can escalate into a sequence of events that concludes with devastating and often deadly results for all involved (Goldstein 1999b; Goldstein, *et al.* 1981).

LITERATURE REVIEW

Violence prevention programmes in schools

Public concern about tragic school violence episodes continues worldwide. Surveys actually demonstrate that violent behaviour, at least among US students, has declined (Coyeman 2000). Researchers have related this progress to a growing awareness of the problem among parents, administrators and teachers (Olweus 1993; Savoye 2000).

Despite this increase in awareness and implementation of school prevention programmes, several theorists believe that children are having difficulty controlling their own behaviour, and recommend interventions which decrease aggressive incidents before they turn into disruptive and violent behaviour (Goldstein 1999b; Goleman 1995; Olweus 1979). According to Goleman (1995), 'the prototypical pathway to violence and criminality starts with children who are aggressive and hard to handle in first and second grade' (p.236). Early attempts at prevention programmes in the schools may be key interventions in the effort to decrease school violence.

Many people have looked at violence prevention methods such as early intervention (Slaby *et al.* 1995) and increasing social skills (Fried and Fried 2003; Goldstein 1999a). Early childhood educators have the opportunity to prevent violence through their modelling of effective interactions with children and others in the classroom. Socialization is defined by Elkin (1960) as a process by which individuals learn to function in society as part of a social group by learning appropriate behaviours, values and feelings that influence how a person behaves within a group. According to Slaby *et al.* (1995) prevention principles are actualized and modelled in the classroom, where children learn that violence can be controlled and prevented. Schools and classrooms may then establish standards and expectations within a group experience by which rules of appropriate behaviours are actualized and a group norm is set.

DANCE MOVEMENT THERAPY AND VIOLENCE PREVENTION IN SCHOOLS

Historically, dance played an integral part in people's lives. The learning about expectations, social norms and values was passed on through dances and story-telling (Primus 1989). The intervention and use of a dance movement therapy process helps individuals learn about and develop their social interactions with others, through modelling of effective interactions with others using movement within a group experience (Sandel and Johnson 1987), as well as providing opportunities for the mastery of movement skills, leading to a sense of self-control (Grabner *et al.* 1999). Fried and Fried state that the lack of basic social skills has caused problems for children and that 'many elementary schools are offering courses on learning how to share, initiating friendships, accepting responsibility for your mistakes, cooperating with a group...' (2003, p.105). There exist many effective violence prevention programmes throughout the US and the world, such as 'Bullyproof Your School' and 'Quit It' (Coyeman 2000).

In the field of dance movement therapy, several violence prevention programmes and training workshops are established. Research studies have been conducted to measure their effectiveness. Dance movement therapist Fried conducts workshops nationally for administrators, teachers, parents and students in order to address issues of school violence such as bullying (Fried and Fried 2003). In Argentina, dance movement therapist Fischman (2005) has addressed issues of violence through dance movement therapy workshops by focusing on improving the empathetic capacities of educators and health professionals. In the US there are several dance movement therapists who are having an impact working with violence prevention in schools. Amongst them, Kornblum (2002) has written about her violence prevention curriculum for elementary school-aged children that was subsequently evaluated with positive results (Hervey and Kornblum 2006). Other research completed in the field has investigated prevention programmes that use an integration of dance/movement, literature and verbalization for bullying prevention in a middle (ages 12 to 15) school (Beardall 1998).

Few studies have evaluated the impact of prevention programmes that model socialization within the group process using dance movement therapy methods to lower aggression problems (Koshland and Whittaker 2004).

THE STUDY

As a dance movement therapist and social worker I developed PEACE through dance movement therapy, a violence prevention programme in an elementary school to address aggression and disruptive behaviours in youth (Koshland and Whittaker 2004). Jean La Sarre Gardner, certified teacher and expressive arts educator, who had studied with me, helped to develop and run the PEACE programme.

A pilot study was designed to match the research in the violence prevention literature which supported the need for lowering aggression before it escalates (Goldstein 1999b) by building pro-social skills (Goldstein 1999a) and by modelling and practising methods of self-control in the PEACE school violence prevention programme. In order to evaluate and measure whether or not the PEACE programme provided methods for building self-control and pro-social behaviours (Goldstein 1999a), I specifically selected and used measurement tools (adapted, with permission, from Goldstein 1999a and Goldstein and Glick 1987) that recorded the number of incidents of positive and negative behaviours reported by multiple data sources collected before and after children received the PEACE programme. Many of the methods for building self-control used in the programme were introduced through children's acquiring physical mastery as they practised a skill such as moving and stopping. The results of studies by Goldstein and Glick (1987) have shown consistently positive effects for adolescents' skill in learning and practising new pro-social behaviours through role-plays involving positive solutions to a variety of relationship conflicts.

Using grant funds from the Marian Chace Foundation of the American Dance Therapy Association, I completed an evaluation of this programme (Koshland and Whittaker 2004).

Aim

This study evaluated the effectiveness of a 12-week dance movement therapy-based violence prevention programme designed to teach skills for building self-control and decreasing aggressive incidents and disruptive behaviours at an elementary school in an urban setting in the Southwest US. The study endeavoured to investigate whether the programme affected how children conducted themselves socially in such a way that aggressive incidents decreased.

Research design

Effectiveness of the programme was evaluated by:

- a between-subjects design that compared aggressive incidents reported to the office for programme participants and non-participants
- a within-subjects design that used pre- and post-measures of behaviour from teachers' perceptions
- a within-subjects design that used pre- and post-measures of children's perceptions of problem behaviours
- a within-subjects design using actual classroom observations before, during and after programme implementation.

The protocol for this dance movement therapy-based violence prevention programme used socialization and engagement of children in a creative, problem-solving group process, introducing pro-social behaviours and methods of self control using dance movement, children's stories and music from different cultures, and discussion (Koshland and Whittaker 2004). The use of a dance movement therapy group which introduced stories and music from different cultures promoted a sense of cultural and community identity when serving children from diverse populations.

Participants

The school population consisted of both immigrants and first-generation Americans. More than half were Spanish-speaking children; around 20 per cent were Caucasian/European; just over 15 per cent were of Native Pacific Island origin; less than 5 per cent were of either Native American or African American children. Eighty-nine per cent of the children were at or below the poverty rate. The five classrooms included: two first grade classes (aged six to seven), one second grade class (aged seven to eight) and two third grade classes (aged eight to nine). A total of 54 children participated in the programme and met for 50 minutes weekly for a period of 12 consecutive weeks. Those classes that did not receive the treatment programme were classes in the fourth, fifth and sixth grades (Koshland and Whittaker 2004).

Five participating classrooms for research were identified in grades one, two and three. The upper level grades were used for comparison of aggressive behaviours as a quasi-control. The administrative requirements for conducting the evaluation through an institutional review board (IRB) were completed; the informed consent forms were gathered; and all other procedural formats were arranged with the principal and school district administration.

The intervention

Dance movement therapy methods used in each programme session aimed to accomplish the programme goals related to socialization (Koshland and Whittaker 2004). Three skill-building areas were introduced over the course of the 12-week programme: (a) self-control, (b) emotional regulation, and (c) problem-solving. The focuses of the sessions were each group's dynamic relational problems and issues around self-control and emotional arousal.

Each of the dance movement therapy methods will be described briefly below, accompanied by the three skill-building areas that were introduced in the PEACE programme.

METHOD A: MOVEMENT OBSERVATION OF THE GROUP'S DYNAMIC AND RANGE OF INTENSITY AND ENERGY LEVEL FOR BUILDING SKILLS OF SELF-CONTROL

Skill building: self-control

Self-control, one of the skill-building areas and methods used, was conceptualized as helping children gain control of their emotions, their physical actions in relation to others, and their problem-solving abilities around peer relationships and social difficulties (Koshland and Whittaker 2004). An example of a dance movement therapy directive intervention used with the children in the programme to help accomplish self-control is 'Let's see if we can go and then stop, by following the leader who stays with the beat of the music.' This process of moving with a set time and focus immediately engaged the children in practising a method of self-control. Other interventions involved listening, self-calming and exploring personal space.

METHOD B: DEVELOPMENT OF CREATIVE EXCHANGES FOR EXPLORATION OF PERSONAL AND SOCIAL SPACE TO INCREASE AWARENESS OF SELF AND OTHER

Skill building: awareness of self and other

In order to further enhance children's focus and control, creative exchanges defining personal and social space, and improvisations related to the story for the session, were used. For example, after reading *The Owl and the Woodpecker*, by Brian Wildsmith, personal space was explored as children were asked to make a shape of a tree that the owl lived in, using their arms, back and whole self to move, going and stopping while remaining in their space. Children were then asked to move through the social space and rearrange their tree shapes made in the forest in a new space by the count of ten. Creative exchanges were allowed to evolve in the movement interactions that occurred between children (Koshland and Whittaker 2004).

METHOD C: DEVELOPMENT OF MOVEMENT STRUCTURES FOR BUILDING SKILLS OF SELF-REGULATION AND CONTROL OF EMOTIONAL AROUSAL

Skill building: emotional regulation

Problems with self-regulation or internal control of emotional arousal were manifest in extreme difficulties with issues of exclusion, and with moving through the space without escalating into disruptive behaviours such as pushing others. One technique to work with regulation problems was the use of a movement structure, 'building a storm', that worked with the concept of acceleration/deceleration combined with imagery from a story about 'angry trees'. Keeping their feet rooted in the ground (remaining in place), children physically practised by increasing their timing, moving (their arms, back, whole self) faster while 'building a storm', and then by decreasing their timing, moving back to slow movement, letting the storm subside (Koshland and Whittaker 2004).

METHODS D AND E: IDENTIFICATION OF EMOTIONAL/SOCIAL AND INTERACTION PROBLEMS FOR BUILDING SKILLS OF DEALING WITH CONFLICTS AND DIFFERENCES IN A NON-AGGRESSIVE MANNER

Skill building: problem-solving and relationships

In each class session, problem-solving was tailored, mainly through movement challenges designed to address difficulties around handling conflicts, peer relations and differences. One intervention that addressed problem-solving was a movement structure called 'Portraits/different solutions'. Children were asked to choose a character to role-play from the bully scene in the story *Angel Child, Dragon Child* by Michelle Maria Surat. Children were asked to find a different solution than bullying. Each group made a decision as to where they wanted to move and stand in relation to others, by changing and moving to a new space on their given count. This movement process developed a dialogue through shapes and being in relation to others in a new way (i.e. witness group stands next to and supports the victims), which generated conversation with one another. This movement structure was intended to expand upon their understanding of communication and problem-solving issues by practising such skills as slowing down before responding, listening and resolving differences without fighting.

Methods of data collection

Several sources were identified for gathering data about the effectiveness of the programme. The children provided one source. Children's responses were collected using the student response form, one week before and one week after completion of the programme. The student response form used a picture-based assessment revised from Goldstein's 'Nonreader's Hassle Log' (1999a) to record children's perceptions of:

1. aggressive incidents that they saw at school (i.e. teasing, fighting, arguing, somebody took something, doing something wrong, throwing something)
2. where the incidents took place at school (i.e. on the playground, cafeteria, gym, bathroom, classroom, office, halls or library)
3. feelings about witnessing the incidents (i.e. happy, OK, sad, mad and scared)
4. how children responded on a feeling level to the incidents witnessed.

Modifications were made to meet a diverse population. This instrument was selected because it used a picture response format that would allow the children's response to be reached independently, and thereby served as a more valid measure (Koshland and Whittaker 2004).

Teachers provided another source of information by completing a behaviour checklist to rate aggressive behaviours for each child, one week before the initiation of the programme and one week after its conclusion, using the behaviour incident report Form A (Goldstein and Glick 1987, by permission). The behaviour incident report Form A is a listing of the negative behaviours only, which is shown in the behaviour incident report Form B (Goldstein and Glick 1987, by permission). (See negative behaviours of behaviour incident report Form B in Table 2.1.)

Changes in the teachers' observation of the children before and after the programme were tested for significance using a dependent t-test measure.

A social work intern for each of the five classes made three random classroom observations pre-, middle, and post-programme completion, and rated the number of pro-social and negative behaviours. The behaviour incident report Form B was a checklist form used. This form was shortened from the original checklist and two items were added for noting the teacher's use of the poems with gestures taught for generalization of skills (see Table 2.1). Poems with gestures were used so that children could transfer prevention skills for focusing when in areas such as the classroom. An example is 'Turn Down the Volume' 'I can work in the quiet zone. Quiet voice, quiet hands, ignore distractions yes I can' (Koshland and La Sarre Gardner 2003).

The last source of information came from the principal's regular log of aggressive incidents that were collected throughout the year. Counts of incidents reported for the participating classrooms in the quarter prior to the programme implementation and the quarter during which the programme was in operation were recorded. Reports for control classrooms that did not receive the programme were also recorded.

Findings and discussion

The results of this pilot study revealed statistically significant decreases in aggression and problem behaviours as noted by children, by teachers and by classroom observations. In addition, a significant difference was noted in the aggressive incidents reported to the principal's office for classrooms that attended the programme, compared to classrooms that did not attend (Koshland and Whittaker 2004).

Students noted significant decreases ($p < .05$) of aggressive behaviours, which included them seeing or experiencing someone doing something wrong or hurtful and someone throwing something (see Table 2.2).

Table 2.1: Behaviour incident report Form B (adapted from Goldstein and Glick 1987, with kind permission of Springer Science and Business Media).

Checklist recording negative and positive behaviours
NEGATIVE BEHAVIOURS
Instigated argument/fight
Threatened, intimidated
Failed to calm down when requested
Became antagonistic when registering a complaint
Argued when told not to
Was short tempered and quick to show anger
Involved in physical fights
Threw articles e.g. pencil, book
Slammed doors, punched walls, kicked objects
POSITIVE BEHAVIOURS
Provided advice, helped others when upset
Expressed self appropriately when frustrated or upset
Expressed feelings appropriately when failed at task
Controlled his or her temper
When failed, was able to try again
Calmed down in a reasonable amount of time when angry
Able to wait when couldn't have his or her way right away
Expressed an opinion different from the group's
Used focusing/listening skills, 'turn down the volume'
Was able to use self-settling skills, 'shifting gears'

Table 2.2: T-tests on changes of aggressive behaviour noted by children

Aggressive behaviour	**t-value**	**df**	**p**
Their seeing or experiencing someone having done something wrong or hurtful	-3.23	53	< .05
Someone throwing something	-3.32	53	< .05

The student response forms on perceptions of problem behaviours were standardized to account for the different numbers of students in each class, and then analysed through a one-tailed dependent measures t-test that showed statistically significant changes (Koshland and Whittaker 2004).

Generally, students noted fewer disruptive behaviours in the different parts of the school observed (see Table 2.3).

Table 2.3: T-tests on changes of behaviour noted by students in different school areas

School areas	t-value	df	p
Bathroom	-1.85	53	< .05
Gym	-2.63	53	< .05
Office	-2.18	53	< .05
Halls	-2.84	53	< .05

The children showed a decrease of feeling 'scared' in handling themselves in aggressive situations ($p < .05$, t-value = -1.77, df = 53) (Koshland and Whittaker 2004).

These observations reported by students suggest that they saw less disruptive behaviour and that they were less scared when handling themselves in problem situations. Such observations reported by students imply that they had gained increased self-control and competency to handle problems, and there was less external disruptive behaviour, either seen or experienced (Koshland and Whittaker 2004). The results of this study regarding students' increased self-control and competency to handle problems and learning about handling relationship conflicts confirm findings and implications from other work that dance movement therapy helps in self-control (Fried and Fried 2003; Grabner *et al.* 1999; Hervey and Kornblum 2006).

Data for teachers' ratings of students were standardized according to a student-to-teacher ratio. These standardized scores were then compared via dependent measures t-tests. Results from these analyses, showing a statistically significant decrease ($p < .05$) of aggressive behaviours as noted by teachers, using the behaviour incident report Form A (Goldstein and Glick 1987, by permission) are presented in Table 2.4.

Table 2.4: T-tests on changes of aggressive behaviour noted by teachers

Aggressive behaviour	t-value	df	p
Children instigating fights	-1.77	53	< .05
Failing to calm down	-1.94	53	< .05
Being upset when couldn't do something immediately	-1.94	53	< .05
Being short-tempered and quick to show anger	-2.20	53	< .05
Being aggravated or abusive when frustrated	-1.70	53	< .05
Being involved in physical fights, and throwing articles	-1.70	53	< .05

These observations reported by teachers suggest that they saw a reduction in disruptive and acting out behaviours in their students, as well as increased capabilities of their students to gain internal control by calming down when upset or frustrated, and by being involved in fewer physical fights. Such observations as reported by teachers, that they saw a reduction in fighting and disruptive behaviours in their students, corresponds to findings from work by Goldstein and Glick (1987) of positive effects for adolescents' skills in learning and practising positive solutions to relationship conflicts, as well as decreasing aggressive incidents behaviour before they turn into violent behaviour (Goldstein 1999b).

Results from the pre-, middle and post-programme classroom observations showed a significant decrease in negative behaviours listed in behaviour incident report Form B. However, there were no significant increases of pro-social positive behaviours found. Prior to examining independent observers' evaluations of classroom behaviour on a question-by-question basis, overall negative and positive evaluations of student behaviour were compared independently. In order to do this, negative classroom behaviours were summed across teacher, and across condition. Pre and post means were then compared for negative behaviours and positive behaviours via dependent measures t-tests. While no change was noted in students' positive behaviours over time, several negative behaviours decreased significantly ($N = 45$, $df = 44$, $p < .001$) (Koshland and Whittaker 2004). These findings reported from the classroom observations of significant decreases in negative behaviours confirm, as suggested by Slaby *et al.* (1995), that violence can be controlled and prevented when prevention principles are modelled in the classroom.

Evidence of decrease in aggressive incidents reported to the office for classrooms before and after the programme was compared with data from those classrooms not involved in the programme. Specifically, the number of incidents reported to the office for treated and untreated students was compared via a Chi square test. There was a statistically significant decrease for those groups that received the treatment, compared to those that did not ($df = 1$, $N = 53$, $\chi^2 = 26.55$, $p < .001$). While data showed a decrease in the number of aggressive incidents reported to the principal for the entire school, the decrease in the number of incidents of treatment groups was significantly greater than the decrease reported in the untreated groups (Koshland and Whittaker 2004).

Overall, it was found that there were significant decreases in aggression and disruptive behaviours as measured by each instrument used. There was not an increase noted in positive or pro-social behaviours (Koshland and Whittaker 2004).

One goal of the design of the dance movement therapy treatment programme was to offer children practice for building positive leadership and peer interactions by structuring their play through movement experiences so that they would acquire skills of self-regulation for less aggressive interactions. These intended acquired skills of children's internal control of their emotions, and their physical actions and interactions in relation to others, could be then transferred and applied in other settings. The random classroom visits showed a significant decrease in the frequency of negative behaviours. This may be a result of students' increased awareness of self-control and problem-solving skills gained in their participation in the dance movement treatment programme and observed by the random classroom observations. Classroom teachers were observed using the generalization poems with hand gestures during every one of the random visits done with each of the five classes rated by the observer. However, data analysis showed that children did not see measurable changes by self-report, or experience less aggression on the playground (Koshland and Whittaker 2004).

The use of measurement tools selected from Goldstein (1999a) and Goldstein and Glick (1987) were effective instruments to measure negative and positive behaviours for violence prevention work, given an easy, short and quick checklist form that included familiar behaviour terms. This provided a user-friendly, applicable tool that has been shown to be a reliable source used by others (Goldstein 1999a; Goldstein and Glick 1987).

Qualitative data findings of the children's perceptions about the programme were done at the end of each group session during discussion and recorded through extensive notes. These data recordings provided information on the children's perspectives on what was working, what were the problems, what was fun and what was helpful about the programme.

Limitations

The limitations of this pilot study lay in the lack of a suitable control group matched with the same age group for comparing those students with and without treatment of a dance movement therapy group. A suitable match and control group for this study would have used first, second and third graders who received the evaluation tools at the same time that the remaining first, second and third graders received both the treatment programme and evaluation tools (Koshland and Whittaker 2004).

Another limitation of this pilot study was the modifications I made to Question 3 and 4 on the student form, so that both used pictures of emotions. This may have been confusing for the students to use, limiting the value of their responses (Koshland and Whittaker 2004).

CONCLUSIONS

The major purpose of the PEACE programme was to decrease aggressive incidents through the intervention of a dance movement therapy group process that introduced methods for building self-control and socialization. The results of this pilot study of the PEACE programme as reported by teachers, by students and by classroom observations demonstrated a significant decrease in aggressive behaviours in several areas as a result of the children's increased ability to control disruptive behaviours such as instigating fights.

This study lays the foundation for further exploration of the use of dance movement therapy to help decrease violence in schools. To further study the intervention, using a second implementation in addition to the PEACE programme could be tested against a method control group of those not receiving the programme, so as to rule out other causes for changes. Further research studies of this intervention should have matched treatment and no-treatment participants in order to have a control group for complete statistical comparisons. From the experience so far, however, it appears that the measurement instruments used in this study (Goldstein 1999a; Goldstein and Glick 1987) can be recommended for use by other dance movement therapists and arts therapists working in schools as a means to verify behavioural changes linked with their particular intervention.

ACKNOWLEDGMENTS

I thank the Marian Chace Foundation of the American Dance Therapy Association for their financial support for this research study; Robyn Flaum Cruz, PhD, research and design consultant; Arnold G. Goldstein, PhD (recently deceased), research supporter and use of instrument tools; J. Wilson B. Whittaker, PhD, research statistician; Douglas Goldsmith, PhD, research consultant; Wendy Dunford, MSW, behaviour observations of research; Jean La Sarre-Gardner, MA in psychology, certified teacher and expressive arts educator, who helped to develop and run the PEACE programme; Sanford Meek, PhD, Joan Lewin, ADTR, dance movement therapist, reader and mentor; Suzi Tortora, EdD, ADTR, CMA, dance movement therapist, and mentor; Julie Miller, principal, and all of the staff and children at the facility where data were collected and for use of materials given with kind permission of Springer Science and Business Media.

REFERENCES

Beardall, N.G. (1998) *Creating a Peaceable School: Confronting Intolerance and Bullying.* MA: Newton Public Schools.

Coyeman, M. (2000) 'Pulling together.' *Christian Science Monitor 92,* 232, 11.

Elkin, F. (1960) *The Child and Society: The Process of Socialization.* New York: Random House.

Fischman, D. (2005) 'La Mejora de la Capaciad Empatica en Profesionales de la Salud y la Education a Traves de Talleres de Danza Movimento Terapia.' ('The Improvement of the

Empathetic Capacity in Health Professionals and Educators through Dance/Movement Therapy Workshops.') Doctoral thesis. Universidad de Palermo, Buenos Aires, Argentina.

Fried, S. and Fried, P. (1996) *Bullies and Victims: Helping Your Child through the Schoolyard Battlefields.* New York: M. Evans and Company Inc.

Fried, S. and Fried, P. (2003) *Bullies, Targets, and Witnesses. Helping Children Break the Pain Chain.* New York: M. Evans and Company Inc.

Goldstein, A.P. (1999a) *The Prepare Curriculum. Teaching Prosocial Competencies.* (Revised edition.) 'Nonreader's Hassle Log' (p. 261). Champaign, IL: Research Press, 261.

Goldstein, A.P. (1999b) *Low-level Aggression: First Steps on the Ladder to Violence.* Champaign, IL: Research Press.

Goldstein, A.P. and Glick, B. (1987) *Aggression Replacement Training. A Comprehensive Intervention for Aggressive Youth.* 'Behaviour Incident Report Form A' (p.318). 'Behaviour Incident Report Form B' (p. 319). Champaign, IL: Research Press.

Goldstein, J.H., Davis, R.W., Kernis, M. and Cohn, E.S. (1981) 'Retarding the escalation of aggression.' *Social Behaviours and Personality 9,* 65–70.

Goleman, D. (1995) *Emotional Intelligence: Why It Can Matter More than IQ.* New York: Bantam Books.

Grabner, T.E., Goodill, S.W., Hill, E.S. and Neida, K.V. (1999) 'Effectiveness of dance/movement therapy on reducing test anxiety.' *American Journal of Dance Therapy 21,* 1, 19–33.

Hervey, L. and Kornblum, R. (2006) 'An evaluation of Kornblum's body-based violence prevention curriculum for children.' *The Arts in Psychotherapy 33,* 2, 113–129.

Kornblum, R. (2002) *Disarming the Playground. Violence Prevention through Movement and Pro-social Skills.* Oklahoma: Wood & Barnes Publishing.

Koshland, L. and Whittaker, J.B. (2004) 'Peace through dance/movement: evaluating a violence prevention programme.' *American Journal of Dance Therapy 26,* 2, 69–90.

Koshland, L. and LaSarre-Gardner, J. (2003) *Peace through Dance/movement Therapy. A Violence Prevention Programme for Elementary School Children.* Self-published educational booklet. Salt Lake City, UT: Lynn Koshland/Self-published.

Olweus, D. (1979) 'Stability of aggressive reaction patterns in males: a review.' *Psychological Bulletin 86,* 852–875.

Olweus, D. (1993) *Bullying at School. What we Know and What we Can Do.* UK/USA: Blackwell Books.

Primus, P. (1989) 'Life Crises: From Birth to Death.' In American Dance Therapy Association: *A Collection of Early Writings: Toward a Body of Knowledge,* 1, 98–110.

Sandel, S.L. and Johnson, D.R. (1987) *Waiting at the Gate: Creativity and Hope in the Nursing Home.* New York: The Haworth Press.

Savoye, C. (2000) 'Violence dips in nation's schools.' *Christian Science Monitor 92,* 141, 1.

Slaby, R.G., Roedell, W.C., Arezzo, D. and Hendrix, K. (1995) *Early Violence Prevention. Tools for Teachers of Young Children.* Washington, DC: National Association for the Education of Young Children.

Surat, M.M. (1983) *Angel Child, Dragon Child.* New York: Scholastic Books.

Wildsmith, B. (1971) *The Owl and the Woodpecker.* Oxford: Oxford University Press.

Chapter 3

Finding a Way out of the Labyrinth through Dance Movement Psychotherapy

Collaborative Work in a Mental Health Promotion Programme in Secondary Schools

Vicky Karkou, Ailsa Fullarton and Susan Scarth

INTRODUCTION

Setting the scene

In the UK at least one in ten children aged 5 to 15 faces emotional, social or behavioural problems such as anxiety, depression, conduct, hyperkinetic and other less common disorders (Office for National Statistics 2004). The same source states that, with the exception of hyperkinetic disorders, rates increase during adolescent years, presenting, overall, a worrying picture of the mental health of young people in Britain.

Although UK government policies acknowledge the need to increase awareness amongst professionals regarding the mental health of children and young people, and to prioritize mental health improvement for this age group (DoH 2004; Scottish Executive 2004), very little appears to have been implemented. Factors such as poor socio-economic family background, long parental unemployment combined with smoking, drinking and cannabis use, youth crime, 'looked after' status and homelessness create a complex picture that is difficult to alter. Increasing suicide rates amongst young people since the 1980s (Office for National Statistics 2004) indicate that, despite government policies, the psychological health of young people remains problematic and implementation of mental health promotion and improvement policies are slow. There are few studies that address the use of the arts therapies in mental health promotion programmes.

In response to this situation, the Labyrinth project has been devised, delivered and evaluated in mainstream secondary schools in England. As we will see in this chapter, the project provides an example of the potential contribution of arts therapies (and dance movement psychotherapy in particular) within a mental health promotion and early intervention context.[3]

LITERATURE REVIEW

Mental health promotion programmes in schools

Secondary education has traditionally been regarded as the cornerstone for enabling the transition of young people from childhood to adult life. Personal, social and health education (PSHE) in England and Wales (Qualifications and Curriculum Authority 2000) and the equivalent Personal and Social Education (PSE) in Scotland (National Qualifications online 2005) is a designated place within the curriculum where emotional/social issues associated with this transition can be addressed. However, educators often feel ill-equipped to deal with emotional issues (Murray 1998) and may feel even more uneasy about dealing with more serious mental health problems (e.g. Rowing and Holland 2000). The Office for Standards in Education (Ofsted) (2005) reveals that increasing pressure on teachers to take into account the emotional and social well-being of their students, combined with a lack of training on mental health issues, means that schools often struggle to address the psychological needs of their pupils.

At the same time, the literature repeatedly reports that the central involvement of educators is crucial for effective school-based programmes (Osborne 2003; Paternite and Johnston 2005). Teachers, by virtue of their

3 The name of the project was inspired from the ancient Greek myth that tells us that the Labyrinth was so artfully constructed that no one could navigate it unaided. After a number of young men and women were killed, Theseus, helped by Ariadne, killed the monster and found his way out of the Labyrinth. The story is used as a metaphor of young people trying to make sense of their lives, but often feeling lost. Unless, like Theseus, they are given help, they can fall victims to the Minotaur.

daily contact with a number of students and the nature of their training, tend to have an understanding of standardized norms and age-appropriate behaviours. Research studies suggest that teachers' observational skills concerning child behaviour are often developed to a much higher standard than those of the parents themselves (Jensen 2000; Porrino *et al.* 1983; Rapoport *et al.* 1986). It is therefore common for school-based prevention programmes to rely on teachers to identify problems, rate problems and report change; at times also to deliver the programmes themselves.

There are a number of different types of mental health promotion programmes in schools. Durlak and Wells (1997), in their meta-analysis of such work in the USA, claim that different programmes can be distinguished by their level of intervention and the way the population is selected. For example, some projects attempt a 'person-centred', others an 'environment-centred' intervention. The former offer direct services to students without attempting changes in the school culture, while in the latter the environment is targeted, in the hope that, by changing the culture, there will be positive effects upon individuals. Regarding the selection of the population, some programmes target all the students (e.g. whole school), others focus upon students at risk, while a third type focuses upon students in transition. Overall, positive change is found for most programmes reviewed, and in particular for those attempting to modify school environments, person-centred mental health promotion programmes and transition programmes. In most cases, both reduction of problems and increase of competences have been observed. Durlak and Wells (1997) also make suggestions for further improvements, including the need for a clear specification of programme goals and content of intervention, and the need to evaluate quality.

A systematic review completed a few years later by Wells *et al.* 2003 adds that positive effects are particularly relevant when a whole-school approach is adopted, the programme is implemented for a whole year, and it aims at mental health promotion rather than mental illness prevention. None of these studies, however, included mental health promotion programmes using the arts therapies.

Psychotherapy and adolescent development

Arts therapists often draw upon psychotherapeutic literature as a way of acquiring in depth understanding of the psychological needs of their clients. Regarding adolescents, a number of different theories can be of particular value. For example, the development of good emotional health in childhood and subsequently in adolescence can often be perceived as closely linked with the attachment process that a child experiences with primary caregivers. Bowlby (1969) was pioneering in this field, and his theory on attachment informs much of the therapeutic work delivered by arts therapists when they work with children and adolescents.

Attachment theory can be explained as a psychological theory about interpersonal human relationships based on the quality of bond that exists between an infant and the primary caregiver, typically the mother (Bowlby 1969). Bowlby argues that the human infant has a need for a secure relationship with adult caregivers, and that without this, normal social and emotional development will be difficult to master. Bowlby (1969) further explains that different relationship experiences can lead to different developmental outcomes. A number of attachment styles with distinct characteristics have been identified in infants. These are known as 'secure', 'avoidant', 'anxious' and 'disorganized' attachment (Ainsworth *et al.* 1978; Bowlby 1969). The last three types listed here refer to maladapted attachment that can often lead to impaired social and emotional development in childhood. An understanding of these types of attachment patterns can shed light to some of the issues pertinent during the transition to adolescence.

Looking at other closely linked perspectives on adolescence, this stage of human development is seen as having particular characteristics and difficulties. For example, Freudian thinking (Freud 1958) regards this period as the time when older, unresolved issues reappear; Winnicott (1965) sees adolescent behaviour as an often unconscious cry for help in resolving past traumas; while Blos (1962) regards this time as one of mourning and loss due to the need to reorganize 'infantile objects' (i.e. infantile internal perceptions of 'significant others' such as parents and other primary caretakers) and to seek autonomy and independence. Erikson (1968) refers to this period as a 'moratorium', i.e. the time when one sheds the childhood ego and explores new ways of being in adulthood, without yet committing to it. The main life issue to overcome is 'identity versus identity confusion'. Past identifications with parents and significant others are questioned, while new attachments and identifications with peers are explored. There is a simultaneous wish to separate from the family and a desperate fear of doing so. Erikson (1968) argues that this stage of 'identity crisis' can be useful and crucial for 'identity formation', but at times it can lead to 'identity diffusion', i.e. the adoption of stereotype identities through joining groups or cliques that often involve rejection of parts of one's self, such as one's ethnicity or sexual identity.

Interestingly, such groups or cliques often evolve around the arts, e.g. in preference for a specific style of music or dance. The arts can therefore be used to reinforce 'stereotype identities'. Paradoxically, the arts may also become an attractive starting point and a useful means of communication for those who may otherwise remain hesitant or unwilling to communicate verbally with adults close to them (McArdle *et al.* 2002). At the same time, given that young people are actively engaged in looking for new relationships and attachments with peers, group work can become particularly relevant to them (Evans 1998).

With groups being an important part of adolescent development, the contribution from the field of group psychotherapy is very useful in furthering our understanding of group dynamics. Yalom (1970) is a key figure in this field, and influential upon the work of arts therapists. His approach to working with groups can be described as a 'here and now' approach where members of a group are encouraged to observe themselves in the therapy group interaction so that they can improve social interaction in their normal lives. This can be a particularly effective way of working with children and young people who often lack the self-reflective skills necessary to do this independently. In Yalom's (1970) view, the therapy group is a microcosm of other social groups, such as families, and even society itself.

In summary, adolescence is a period of significant cognitive, social and behavioural transitions. There are huge gains in developing cognitive reasoning and acquiring new perspectives, as well as achieving deeper emotional understanding. Socially, peer relationships grow in intensity and become much more important than before. Physically, puberty sparks massive hormonal and physical changes. These developmental changes that begin in early adolescence gradually lead to a desire for a separate identity with concomitant independence and autonomy (Erikson 1968). These transitions are challenging for even the most emotionally well adapted youngsters, and can be even more so for young people who have experienced attachment difficulties in some form. Because of these difficulties, the contribution of interventions such as arts therapies, that enable engagement and non-threatening exploration of emotional and social issues, can be of particular value.

The contribution of arts therapies

According to national figures (Karkou 1998; Karkou and Sanderson 2006) over 60 per cent of registered arts therapists practising in the UK work with children and adolescents. Research evidence suggests that arts therapies can be particularly effective with children and adolescents (e.g. McArdle *et al.* 2002; McQueen 1975), especially when choosing an eclectic, psychodynamic or humanistic approach over a behavioural one (Gold, Voracek and Wigram 2004). Furthermore, dance movement psychotherapy research evidence suggests that this intervention can contribute towards increased vitality, improved body image, stabilizing the sympathetic nervous system, improving psychological distress, and reducing or even alleviating depression (Groenlund *et al.* 2006; Jeong *et al.* 2005; Koch, Morlinghaus and Fuchs 2007; Ritter and Low 1996).

Clinical papers describing how arts therapies work with adolescents (e.g. Emunah 1995; Linesch 1988; Riley 1999) discuss the need to offer space for role experimentation, while others (Jennings and Gersie 1987; Payne 1992a) highlight the need to address adolescent defences such as boredom, absence/lethargy, high anxiety, dependency and self-consciousness.

Clear theoretical understanding and clinical strategies are considered important skills for safe practice with this client group. Links with psychotherapeutic literature are identified in most cases as an aid for understanding adolescent difficulties (Blos 1962; Bowlby 1969; Erikson 1968; Winnicott 1965).

Arts therapists often work in schools with children and adolescents. Pioneers in music, art, drama and dance movement therapy have reported work in these settings (Alvin 1975; Jennings 1987; Nordoff and Robbins 1971; Payne 1992b; Waller 1991), while national statistics suggest that education is the second most common working environment amongst arts therapists and the first amongst dance movement psychotherapists (Karkou and Sanderson 2000, 2001, 2006). Although there is a longer tradition of arts therapists working in special schools, mainstream education is also gaining ground amongst arts therapists (Karkou and Sanderson 2006). When arts therapists work in mainstream schools, it is possible that they engage in mental health promotion activities. However, with few exceptions (Karkou and Glasman 2004), limited published information is available regarding such work.

This chapter attempts to address this issue by presenting selected findings from the evaluation of the Labyrinth project, a mental health promotion programme delivered in mainstream secondary education. Particular attention will be paid to process and outcome findings relating to the work completed with one young person participating in the school-based arts therapies group intervention.

THE STUDY

Aim and objectives

The current project was based on earlier pilot work (Karkou and Glasman 2004; Karkou and Jones 2003; Karkou, Dubowski and Jones 2004) and aimed to promote and improve the mental health of young people in secondary schools through the use of arts therapies.[4] More specifically, the objectives of the project were:

1. to raise awareness amongst teaching staff about issues relating to mental health pertinent to adolescents and the use of arts therapies with this client group
2. to improve the emotional and social well-being of these young people.

In order to meet the objectives set out, a two part-programme was developed that consisted of:

Part A: educational programme for teaching staff that aimed to raise awareness of mental health issues and educate participants on the potential value of arts therapies for troubled young people

Part B: direct group intervention with young people; in this case direct intervention was through a brief (ten sessions) dance movement psychotherapy group, that aimed to increase young people's understanding of mental health issues and contribute towards their emotional and social well-being.

Design

A thorough evaluation was completed for the two parts of the programme, following a mixed design, as Figure 3.1 shows.

Part A (the educational programme) was primarily evaluated post-delivery by participating teachers from three schools completing evaluation forms. Part B followed a randomized controlled trial (RCT) design with dance movement psychotherapy as the group intervention and a waiting list that acted as the control group. Students from one of the three schools were randomly allocated to the two groups.

4 Both the pilot and this study were funded by the Calouste Gulbenkian Foundation.

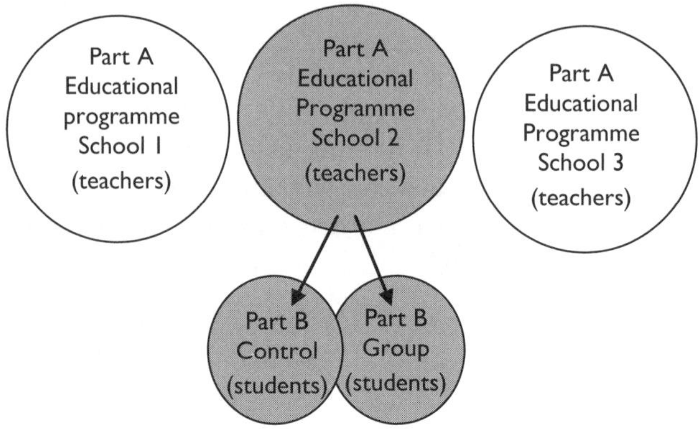

Figure 3.1: Project design

Both quantitative and qualitative data were collected in all cases. More specifically, we used the following methods of data collection:

- ongoing reflective notes/journal completed by teachers, students and therapist
- video recordings of all group sessions with students
- evaluation forms completed by teachers and students
- a 'personal shield' (a measurement of knowledge, skills and attitudes specifically designed for the project, that was completed by participating teaching staff and students)
- the Achenbach System of Empirically Based Assessment (ASEBA) (Achenbach 1991) was a battery of standardized questionnaires that consisted of a 'youth self-report' completed by all the young people participating in the project (both intervention and control groups), a 'teacher's report form' completed by teachers and a 'child behaviour checklist' completed by parents. In all cases, data were collected before and after the intervention (Part B).

The Labyrinth intervention

The two parts of the programme were designed and delivered in a flexible manner as follows.

PART A: EDUCATIONAL PROGRAMME FOR TEACHING STAFF

This was four hours long and consisted of brief presentations, seminar work and workshops for teaching staff. All four hours were delivered within one term in each of the three schools participating in the study. The programme covered: (1) issues of mental health (signs and aetiology of poor mental health, mental health diagnoses and additional educational support); and (2) an introduction to arts therapies (principles underpinning the arts therapies; the role of the arts therapies in supporting school-aged children) and to dance movement psychotherapy in particular.

This stage, broadly speaking, intended to have a whole-school environmental character; Durlak and Wells (1997) have alternatively designated this type of work as an 'ecological' or 'system-level' intervention. Because of the short duration of this intervention, in-depth work did not take place, and so we did not expect significant and/or lasting changes in the whole-school culture. We did expect, however, that teaching staff participating in the study would achieve an increased awareness of mental health issues and a deeper understanding of arts therapies (Objectives 1). It was also hoped that the work completed during this stage would facilitate the selection of one school for the second stage of the project and, once agreements with the school were made, support the smooth running of this second part of the project.

PART B: GROUP INTERVENTION WITH STUDENTS

The dance movement psychotherapy group aimed to develop an understanding among young people about mental health issues, and primarily to improve the emotional and social well-being of these young people (Objective 2). It ran for ten sessions over a school term. Each session was 45 minutes long and consisted of: (1) warm-up activities, (2) theme development, (3) cool-down and (4) reflection/closure.

The work was influenced primarily by dance movement therapists such as Chace (Chaiklin and Schmais 1986), one of the pioneers of dance movement psychotherapy with continuing impact on contemporary practice, and by interpersonal group psychotherapists such as Yalom (1970).[5])

5 Karkou and Sanderson (2006) discuss historical and conceptual links between these two therapists. In conclusion they refer to Chace's approach as an 'interactive/interpersonal' approach that shares a number of principles with Yalom's (1970) interpersonal philosophy. Influences from these two sources were therefore seen as complementary.

In addition, research evidence was taken into account (Gold *et al.* 2004; Groenlund *et al.* 2006; Jeong *et al.* 2005; Koch *et al.* 2007; McArdle *et al.* 2002; Ritter and Low 1996), next to explanations of adolescent development found in psychotherapeutic literature (Bowlby 1969; Blos 1962; Erikson 1968; Winnicott 1965) and clinical suggestions made by arts therapists (Emunah 1995; Jennings and Gersie 1987; Linesch 1988; Riley 1999) and dance movement psychotherapists in particular (Payne 1992a).

The protocol adopted for the specific intervention was designed prior to the commencement of the work and is summarized as follows.

1. Beginnings: building a group
   - establishing group rules and warm-up activities
   - improving self-awareness and getting to know others
   - establishing concentration and communication
   - developing co-operation and problem sharing.
2. Middle: coping strategies
   - learning to protect oneself
   - identifying stressful situations
   - building trust and developing relationships
   - addressing feelings such as loneliness, fear, anger and loss.
3. End: getting help
   - exploring ways of getting help
   - asking for help.

Particularly useful for the translation of theoretical principles to movement were techniques introduced by Chace (Chaiklin and Schmais 1986), as well playful activities developed by Veronica Sherborne (2001) that encourage active relationship building with 'self' and 'other'. Activities introduced in the group sessions reflect these influences. Examples include:

- introduction of movement that reflects introduction of gestures and whole body movements that reflect the mood of the group and individuals within it.

- mirroring and attuning to participants' movement
- building a common rhythm

(all the above are influences from Chace)

- using large cloths to hold, support, enclose and pull along – 'caring' relationships
- using props for creating safe spaces and devising team games as ways in which to foster 'sharing' relationships, i.e. relationships amongst peers with equal power
- exploring safe boundaries, saying 'no!' and experiencing safe and playful 'against' relationships

(the last three examples reflect influences from Sherborne).

The following were also used:

- art-based activities e.g. drawing own body outline, engaging in a group drawing
- drama-based activities, such as role-playing how to deal with difficult situations, enacting 'feeling' words, enacting the story of the Labyrinth.

Throughout the delivery of the work, and when reflecting on the movement dynamics of the individuals and the group (e.g. by analysing video recordings), Laban's (1960) system of movement observation and analysis was utilized.[6]

Participants

PART A: TEACHING STAFF

For the first, educational part of the project, teachers and teaching staff were invited to participate. Particular emphasis was placed on involving Special Educational Needs Co-ordinators (SENCO), teaching staff with specific pastoral duties (year tutors and teachers responsible for PSHE), arts and sports teachers and other personnel with close contact with students (for example, in one school the receptionist participated and in another the school counsellors took part).

---

6 Laban developed a comprehensive system of movement analysis that looks at qualitive aspects of movement.

PART B: STUDENTS

Early adolescents (11-13-year-olds) who, according to the SENCO and year tutors, were at risk of developing mental health problems, participated in this second stage of the work. Inclusion criteria were:

- scholastic under-performance
- known major family problem/s
- malnourishment or poorly cared for appearance
- impaired peer relationships
- presentation of behavioural or emotional difficulties that were not severe enough to require the involvement of specialized mental health services.

Students who were already receiving additional support and/or were being seen by other mental health professionals were excluded from the sample.

Findings and discussion

PART A: SOME FINDINGS FROM THE EDUCATIONAL PROGRAMME

Twenty-one teachers and other teaching staff from three schools participated in the study. Preliminary analysis of data collected through the 'personal shield' completed before the delivery of the programme showed that on a rating scale from 1 to 5 (1 was 'very good' and 5 was 'very poor') participants regarded their knowledge of mental health issues as average (mean = 3.25, standard deviation (SD) = 1.39). This finding was not a surprise, given that several of the participants were working in their schools in pastoral roles (e.g. SENCO, student learning mentor and student welfare officer), and so were expected to have some understanding of their students' mental health issues. In contrast, participants regarded their knowledge of arts therapies as poor (mean = 3.75, SD = 1.28). Again, given that arts therapies do not have an established place within the school system (Karkou 1999; Karkou and Sanderson 2000, 2001, 2006), and that there are few publications that describe the work that is already taking place (Karkou and Glasman 2004), the limited knowledge reported by teaching staff was expected.

In the open-ended questions from the personal shield, participants expressed concerns about whether schools were able, and appropriately equipped, to address mental health issues. The reviewed literature acknowledges this (Murray 1998; Rowing and Holland 2000). Other respondents remarked that mental health issues in children and young people appear to be on the increase, and one participant noted that she felt that mental health issues were 'increasing at an alarming rate'. A similarly alarming picture is presented in the literature (Office for National Statistics 2004), especially regarding the increase in suicide rates amongst young people, and young men in particular. Finally, participants expressed concern that resources for children and young people facing mental health issues were limited, referrals were difficult to make, and waiting lists for specialized services such as Child and Adolescent Mental Health Services were particularly long.

Evaluation forms completed by teaching staff by the end of the delivery of the programme suggested that the majority of the participants regarded the mental health components of the programme as good (mean = 2.10, SD = .73 on a 5-point rating scale from 1 = very good to 5 = very poor), and the introduction to arts therapies as very good (mean = 1.60, SD = .89). Participants also indicated that two of the strengths of the project were the discussion around mental health theories and the experiential components of the work. Although they felt that more time was needed for the delivery of this part of the programme, they also found that presenters complemented each other very well. (The educational programme was delivered by Susan Scarth, the third author of this chapter, who is a dance movement psychotherapist and an art therapist experienced in working with young people.) Participants raised concern about the use of the term 'mental health' as carrying stigma that would hinder co-operation from parents. This concern was addressed by replacing the term 'mental health' with 'well-being' and inserting this in all relevant documentation disseminated to students and their parents.

PART B: SOME FINDINGS FROM THE GROUP INTERVENTION

Twelve students were involved in the second part of the study; six of them were randomly allocated to the dance movement psychotherapy group, while the other six comprised the waiting list that acted as the control group. On the whole, members of the dance movement psychotherapy group showed improvement in relation to a number of the measures used in this second part of the project.

For example, findings from the personal shield revealed that there was an overall improvement in pupils' attitude towards people with emotional difficulties, as well as in terms of their ability to deal with stressful situations. On completion of the intervention, participants evaluated their experience as good (mean = 1.83, SD = .98). They also commented that being with other students was the most enjoyable part of the work. One student remarked that the group 'worked together to achieve more'. The need of adolescents to engage in peer groups has already been discussed in the literature (e.g. Erikson 1968; Evans 1998; McArdle *et al.* 2002). Several participants also commented on their engagement in arts activities as particularly valuable. One pupil remarked, 'I liked doing the activities and doing dance and drama.' This is in accordance with the arts therapies literature that highlights the role of the arts as particularly valuable for adolescents as a means of engagement and role experimentation (Emunah 1995; Linesch 1988; Riley 1999). When the participants were asked what they enjoyed least about the project, all six commented on arguments and bad behaviour of others. One commented that the most annoying thing for her was the 'silliness of people, including me'. It appears that these comments referred to adolescent defences, such as described by Payne (1992a) and Jennings and Gersie (1987). However, the destructive aspects of the work did not detract from participants' valuing their experience in the group. Additional comments included statements such as 'I'm going to miss it' and 'wish I could do it again'.

Results from non-parametric testing performed on the data (paired Wilcoxon test for two groups and Friedman test for more than two groups) are shown in Table 3.1 and indicate that there were a number of statistically significant differences between groups and times, particularly associated with scores from the teacher's report form. These results indicate that teachers completing this standardized questionnaire perceived 'internalizing' behaviour (e.g. anxiety, withdrawal and somatic complaints of the students participating in the dance movement psychotherapy group) as reducing after the intervention, in comparison to the waiting list control group. This is consistent with previous studies that provide evidence that dance movement psychotherapy can reduce anxiety or depression (Groenlund *et al.* 2006; Jeong *et al.* 2005; Koch *et al.* 2007; Ritter and Low 1996;). Reduction of 'internalizing' behaviour also seemed to have an effect on the total scores for the same measure, confirming similarly positive results reported in previous studies (McArdle *et al.* 2002). In the Labyrinth study statistically significant reduction of scores for the 'internalizing' behaviour in the dance movement psychotherapy group also appeared to be true for all the measures used (see Table 3.1).

Table 3.1: Statistically Significant Differences between Groups and Times (Wilcoxon test for two groups and Friedman test for more than two groups)

Type of Measure	Intervention	Scores Before and After Intervention (Time 1 and Time 2)
All measures		
'Internalizing'**	Dance Movement Psychotherapy Group**	Decrease
	Waiting List Group**	Increase
'Externalizing'	Dance Movement Psychotherapy Group	Increase
	Wating List Group	Decrease
Total*	Dance Movement Psychotherapy Group**	Decrease
	Waiting List Group**	Decrease
Teacher's report form		
'Internalizing'**	Dance Movement Psychotherapy Group**	Decrease
	Waiting List Group**	Decrease
'Externalizing'	Dance Movement Psychotherapy Group	Decrease
	Wating List Group	Increase
Total*	Dance Movement Psychotherapy Group**	Decrease
	Waiting List Group**	The same
Youth self-report		
'Internalizing'	Dance Movement Psychotherapy Group	Decrease
	Waiting List Group	Decrease
'Externalizing'	Dance Movement Psychotherapy Group	Increase
	Wating List Group	Decrease
Total	Dance Movement Psychotherapy Group	The same
	Waiting List Group	Decrease

* Accepted as $p < .05$ level of significance
** Accepted at $p <. 01$ level of significance

It is interesting that, based on the teacher's assessment of change, 'externalizing' scores (aggressive and rule-breaking behaviour) remained largely the same (with a minor reduction after the intervention). Given that the use of the arts is often seen as encouraging students to act out, this finding is particularly positive.

In contrast, the scores obtained from the youth self-report demonstrate that young people themselves saw an increase in their 'externalizing' behaviour after the intervention, while their 'internalizing' scores were largely the same. Although these results were not accepted as statistically significant, it is worth noting that possibly as a result of the intervention, young people felt that they were more able to speak out and acknowledge their issues. Often these shifts were made within the 'normal' range of scores. This meant that young people saw their behaviour changing in an outwards fashion, but without becoming inappropriate.

Data collected from parents were incomplete (8 out of 12 parents returned the child behaviour checklist), and because of this and the small overall numbers, results are not discussed here.

In the following section some of the changes described above will be illustrated through the example of Aaron, one of the participants of the dance movement psychotherapy group.

The case of Aaron

Aaron (his name has been changed to protect anonymity) was referred to the group because his year tutor had concerns about his overall mental health. For example, in the teacher's report form his year tutor reported that Aaron presented with primarily 'internalizing' problems, with scores for both anxiety and withdrawn behaviour falling within clinical levels. Aaron was also seen as having social problems, and at times limited attention skills. 'Externalizing' scores remained at normal levels.

The youth self-report completed by Aaron himself indicated that he internalized issues to a pathological degree, while his 'externalizing' behaviour was borderline. More specifically, he presented borderline anxiety, clinical levels for withdrawn behaviour and somatic complaints, and serious thought problems.

Beginnings – Sessions 3 and 4

Aaron missed the first two sessions of the group. When he arrived in Session 3 he engaged immediately, but with a sense of distance. The dance movement psychotherapist noted that he 'seemed older than the other members' (reflective notes). Video analysis of this session shows that in movement he presented himself with a concave shaping in his torso, giving a sense of retreating and self-protection. He seemed to 'give in' to gravity, presenting reduced Strong Weight moving towards Passive Weight Effort (Laban's 1960 terminology) with low energy level – characteristics often associated with the movement profile of people with depression (Stanton-Jones 1992). Despite these features, his head jutted forward and his eye contact was intense, suggesting interest in the group, while his long hair flopped into his eyes, giving him a 'cool' adolescent air. Although he entered the group late and was relatively quiet in the first sessions, he appeared fully alert and aware of his peers, taking a keen interest in the group interactions.

By Session 4, members were exploring personal boundaries within the group by drawing the outline of their bodies on a large piece of paper. Aaron 'drew a tiny figure on his huge piece of paper' (dance movement psychotherapist's reflective notes). Furthermore, the therapist remarked on her sense of being present in front of very young children who were playing alongside each other, not yet able to form meaningful and sustained attachments. Although the task was introduced to offer them an opportunity to build a sense of belonging to the group, according to the dance movement psychotherapist: 'No one can share their space in case they get lost. Aaron seems to have already lost himself!' (reflective notes).

Middle group – Sessions 5–7

As the sessions progressed, Aaron engaged in the group in a number of ways. For example, he was quite energized in the first session following the school's week holiday, but by the sixth session the therapist reported that 'he is disconnected, fragmented in his body – unable to think' (reflective notes). There was a lively theme of 'absent fathers', but Aaron remained quiet – the therapist noted: 'I am particularly touched by what he was *not* saying' (reflective notes). His body shape remained concave and retreating. The one person he connected positively with was Timmy, another group member of particularly small stature.

Aaron's favourite movement during this period involved a 'body popping' right arm movement that was jerky and disconnected from the rest of his body. He repeated this arm movement several times in Session 5, and the therapist wondered if this also indicated a sense of detachment, both within himself and from the group. It is possible that this movement also encapsulated problematic attachment patterns with his peers outside the group and with his family (Bowlby 1969).

During an earlier session, a group member commented on Aaron's poor personal hygiene. He was indeed unkempt, appeared unwashed and had strong body odour. Following that session Aaron attended all group sessions 'washed and clean clothed' (dance movement psychotherapist's reflective notes). The therapist believed this change to be in direct response to the group member's comment. According to Yalom (1970), during the early stages of a group, members deal with finding their way 'in' or 'out' of the group. Paying attention to his personal hygiene in subsequent sessions was possibly Aaron's expression of a wish to be accepted in the group.

As the group progressed Aaron grew in confidence. He welcomed the introduction of cloth props and enjoyed the opportunity to wrap and cover himself up. Meanwhile, his alliance with Timmy continued, with both of them engaging in a country-dance sequence that was energetic and very well co-ordinated. Aaron's relationships with other group members improved as he played a supporting role for a theatrical enactment by one of the girl members, and engaged in another group enactment that explored the theme of Labyrinth. The use of props and symbolic material enabled Aaron to experiment and ultimately form relationships in ways that became less threatening for himself, as well as for the other members of the group.

Props are often perceived within the arts therapies literature as representing what Winnicott (1965) refers to as the 'transitional object' that can be seen as a bridge between the self and other. Both role experimentation and the need for peer connection are extensively discussed in the arts therapies literature with regard to adolescence, and are potentially relevant to Aaron's use of his time within the dance movement psychotherapy group sessions (Emunah 1995; Evans 1998; Linesch 1988; McArdle *et al.* 2002; Riley 1999).

Ending – Sessions 8–10

During this last period, Aaron engaged well when the ground rules were reviewed and a group picture was drawn by all participants. He drew a picture of 'chaos' that gave a sense of him occupying a larger part of the paper than he had done in earlier drawings. He gave the same sense of a 'larger presence' in the group as a whole. This possibly reflects research evidence about the value of dance movement psychotherapy in improving body image and increasing vitality (Koch *et al.* 2007; Ritter and Low 1996). His relationship with Timmy grew, while he continued to engage with other group members. In the penultimate session, which turned out to be the final one for all except one pupil, because of a school trip, Aaron showed that he was both 'able to be pulled [in the cloth] and to pull others' (therapists reflective notes). This suggested that he had found a way to feel contained within the group and able to offer and receive support. At the end of Session 8 Aaron sought some one-to-one time with the therapist, offering to help clear up the room while sharing some personal information about his home life. This was an important moment for Aaron to seek help for himself.

As video analysis shows, Aaron's movements became more integrated, with an increase in connectivity between parts of the body, less concave shaping in his chest, and a more integrated sense of the flow of energy through his body (Laban 1960). The therapist wrote in her final reflection: 'Aaron had engaged well and utilized his time well', and 'the whole ten sessions seemed to be focused on the theme of identity' (reflective notes). On reflection this was certainly Aaron's main theme, as he appeared to become more connected with the group and himself by the end of the sessions.

In the youth self-report completed by Aaron after the intervention, all scores, with the exception of those relating to rule-breaking behaviour, indicate an improvement (see Figure 3.2). This was particularly obvious in the 'internalizing' scores for anxiety, withdrawn behaviour and somatic complaints, which shifted from borderline and clinical levels to normal and borderline levels respectively. A major improvement was also reported regarding thought problems.

It is worth noting that even in the case of rule-breaking behaviour, where the score was higher after the intervention, it remained at normal levels. It is possible that the higher score in rule-breaking behaviour is the result of Aaron becoming more able to externalize issues and speak out, and as such he might have perceived himself to be 'naughty'.

Global scores relating to Aaron's youth self-report after the intervention also showed that there was a major positive shift relating to both 'internalizing' and 'externalizing' problems. More important, overall

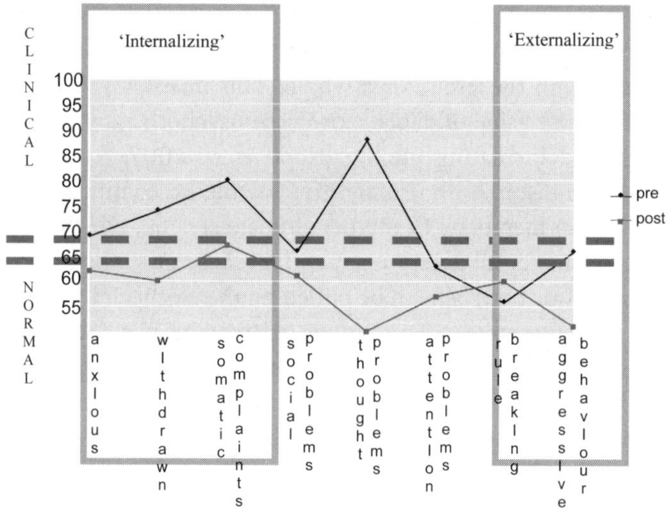

Figure 3.2: Aaron's specific scores from youth self-report

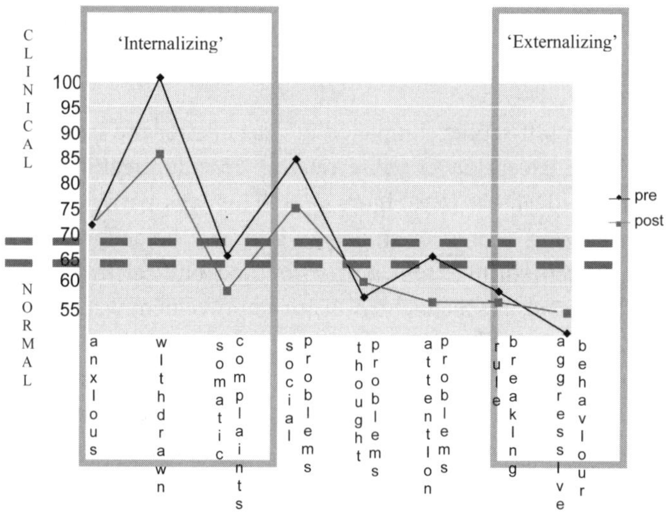

Figure 3.3: Aaron's specific scores from teacher's report form

scores showed that there was a shift from clinical (t-score = 73) to normal levels (t-score = 59).

In the teachers' report form, Aaron's year tutor regarded his behaviour as having improved after the intervention. Although, in this measure, 'internalizing' problems remained at clinical levels, the teacher observed a positive change. Aaron's behaviour was seen as slightly more externalized, but remained at normal levels (see for example, the slightly higher score for aggressive behaviour after the group, in comparison to the score for the same issues before the group presented, in Figure 3.3).

It appeared that although a number of problems remained, scores from the teacher's report form indicated clear improvement in Aaron's behaviour.

CONCLUSIONS

From the findings presented here it seems that, to a large extent, the objectives of the project were met. For example, regarding the educational programme, teaching staff valued the mental health content of the programme that aimed to raise awareness around adolescent difficulties, and valued even more the introduction to arts therapies that aimed to inform participants of therapeutic interventions that could address these difficulties.

Opportunities for discussion in the mental health section, and the experiential components of the arts therapies sessions, were highly regarded. It seemed that the interactive components of the work enabled participants to digest information and acquire a deeper understanding of the issues dealt with. It is possible that this part of the project contributed towards a whole-school approach, which is highly recommended by Wells *et al.* (2003) as contributing towards successful interventions in mental health promotion in schools. Furthermore, it is also possible that by raising awareness around mental health issues and the contribution of arts therapies in the emotional lives of young people, it made the second part of the project easier to introduce. This point ties in with what often takes place when a new service is introduced. Although it is often normal practice amongst arts therapists working on a freelance basis, and/or in short contracts, to offer introductory programmes and workshops to members of staff, this preliminary aspect has not been sufficiently discussed or studied. Practitioners are often inventing and reinventing the wheel. Longer-term awareness-raising interventions are needed, such as might lead to the development of associated introductory packs available to practitioners working in schools.

During the group intervention, young people participating in dance movement psychotherapy commented on the value of working with other students. Feedback from other group members appeared important and powerful – maybe more so than feedback from the therapist. This is evident in the case of Aaron, who, soon after another group member's comments on his unkempt appearance, returned to all following sessions clean and tidy. Because of the need for peer relationships, the value of group work with adolescents that enables honest and respectful interaction between members should not be underestimated.

Other important aspects of the work, as reported by participating students, were their engagement in the arts activities. In this case dance and drama enactments were particularly valued. The case example also brought to the foreground the need for clear ground rules and structure. There was an expectation that the group could easily dissolve into chaos, reflecting the chaotic feelings present in the young people, and the value of a strong theoretical understanding of adolescent development. In a transient art form such as dance, the use of props and dramatic structures for role experimentation and relationship formation can be of great value. Dance movement therapy, in this particular project, appeared to offer opportunities for participants to grow in confidence, improve their body image, develop a sense of relationship and caring for others, and increase their vitality. The use of rhythm, pertinent in Chacian work, might have contributed to the sense of vitality, as well as group cohesiveness and awareness of 'other'. The participants' self-reports of the benefits gained from the intervention supported existing literature stating the value of dance movement psychotherapy for addressing depressive features. This was statistically supported by the teachers' reports, in which overall 'internalizing' behaviours were seen as reduced.

The presence of a control group can offer support for the validity of these findings. However, there was no follow-up to determine the degree to which long-lasting effects were present (due to a change of circumstances in the research team). This, combined with the very small number of participants, does not allow us to generalize from the findings about the effect of this type of intervention on adolescents at risk of developing mental health problems. It does, however, call for further research in the area.

Furthermore, the specific project raises a few important points:

1. The need to spend sufficient time informing teachers about mental health issues and the arts therapies, receiving information from teachers about student issues, family backgrounds and presenting difficulties during normal school time. Strong collaboration with teachers is essential for maximizing therapeutic benefits for the young people involved.
2. The need to engage in evidence-based and theory-informed practice in our work in schools which is tailored around the needs of young people. This becomes even more relevant to this challenging client group.
3. The potential contribution of a range of different methods to evaluate arts therapies, ranging from standardized measures to reflective journals: by using different methods of evaluation, different aspects of the work are highlighted and a more thorough picture is described.
4. Finally, the project highlights the value of collaborative work with other arts therapists. A call for collaborative work has already been made in previous publications (Karkou 2002, 2003) and revisited in the conclusion of this book. The collaboration that has been described here took place between art and dance movement psychotherapists who, during the process of the project, undertook a number of diverse roles such as project co-ordinator, teacher, research assistant and therapist. As arts therapists often work in isolation, coming together in a team was a refreshing experience for us. The project offered a unique opportunity for us to learn from each other, refine our thinking, and further develop our therapeutic and research skills. Collaborative work of this kind within the arts therapies has great potential benefits, and further exploration in this direction could involve professionals from other disciplines – for example, teachers, educational psychologists, health professionals, psychiatrists, researchers, etc. It could also be of particular value to troubled young people, who may benefit from a range of professionals working well together to support them to 'kill the Minotaur' and guide them out of the 'Labyrinth'.

REFERENCES

Achenbach, T. (1991) *Manual for the Teacher's Report Form and 1991 Profile.* Burlington, VT: University of Vermont Department of Psychiatry.

Ainsworth, M., Blehar, M.C., Waters, E. and Wall, S. (1978) *Patterns of Attachment: a Psychological Study of the Strange Situation.* Hillsdale, NJ: Erlbaum.

Alvin, J. (1975) *Music Therapy.* London: John Clare Books.

Blos, P. (1962) *On Adolescence.* New York: The Free Press.

Bowlby, J. (1969) *Attachment and Loss (Vol. 1).* London: Basic Books.

Chaiklin, S. and Schmais, D. (1986) 'The Chace Approach to Dance Therapy.' In P. Lewis (ed.) *Theoretical Approaches in Dance/Movement Therapy, Vol 1.* Dubuque, IA: Kendall/Hunt.

Department of Health (DoH) (2004) *Choosing Health: Intelligence on Mental Health.* Public Health White Paper. Available at www.dh.gov.uk/en/Publichealth/Choosinghealth/DH_072525 accessed on 08 October 2009.

Durlak, J.A. and Wells, A.M. (1997) 'Primary prevention mental health programmes for children and adolescents: a meta-analytic review.' *American Journal of Community Psychology 25,* 2, 115–152.

Emunah, R. (1995) 'From Adolescent Trauma to Adolescent Drama: A Group Drama Therapy with Emotionally Disturbed Youth.' In J. Jennings (ed.) *Dramatherapy with Children and Adolescents.* London: Routledge, 150–169.

Erikson, E. (1968) *Identity, Youth and Crisis.* London: Faber and Faber.

Evans, K. (1998) 'Shaping experience and sharing meaning: art therapy for children with autism.' *Inscape 3,* 1, 17–25.

Freud, A. (1958) 'Adolescence.' *Psychoanalytic Study of the Child 13,* 255–278.

Gold, C., Voracek, M. and Wigram, T. (2004) 'Effects of music therapy for children and adolescents with psychopathology: a meta-analysis.' *Journal of Child Psychology and Psychiatry 46,* 6, 1054–1063.

Groenlund, E., Renck, B. and Vaboe, N.G. (2006) 'How depressed teenage girls can be helped by dance movement therapy.' Presentation in 2nd International Research Colloquium in Dance Therapy, Pfarzheim, Germany.

Jennings, S. (1987) (ed.) *Dramatherapy: Theory and Practice 1.* London and New York: Routledge.

Jennings, S. and Gersie, A. (1987) 'Dramatherapy with Disturbed Adolescents.' In S. Jennings (ed.) *Dramatherapy: Theory and Practice 1.* London and New York: Routledge.

Jensen, P. (2000) 'Commentary.' *Journal of the American Academy of Child and Adolescent Psychiatry 39,* 984–987.

Jeong, Y.J., Hong, S.C., Lee, M.C., Kim, Y.K and Suh, C.M. (2005) 'Dance/movement therapy improves emotional responses and modulates neurohormones in adolescents with mild depression.' *International Journal of Neuroscience 115,* 12, 1711–1720.

Karkou, V. (1998) 'A descriptive evaluation of the practice of arts therapies in the UK.' Unpublished PhD thesis, University of Manchester, School of Education.

Karkou, V., (1999) 'Art therapy in education: findings from a nation-wide survey in art therapies', *Inscape: The Journal of the BAAT, 4,* 2, 62–70.

Karkou, V. (2002) 'Book review: L. Kossolapaw, S. Scoble and D. Waller (eds) *Arts-Therapies-Communication: On a Way to a Communicate European Arts Therapy* (Volume 1).' *Inscape 7,* 1, 43–45.

Karkou, V. (2003) 'New in Print.' L. Kossolapaw, S. Scoble and D. Waller (eds) *Arts-Therapies-Communication: On a Way to a Communicate European Arts Therapy (Volume 1).* Muster, Hamburg, Berlin and London, *E-motion: Association of Dance Movement Therapy UK Quarterly XIV,* 4, 11–13.

Karkou, V. and Jones, (2003) 'The Beginnings of the Labyrinth Project in Secondary Schools.' In N. Govas (ed.) *Proceedings of the 3rd International Theatre and Drama Education Conference: Building Bridges.* Athens, Greece. (In English and Greek)

Karkou, V., Dubowski, J. and Jones, P. (2004) Unpublished project report submitted to the Calouste Gulbenkian Foundation. University of Hertfordshire.

Karkou, V. and Glasman, J. (2004) 'Arts, education and society: the role of the arts in promoting the emotional well-being and social inclusion of young people.' *Support for Learning 19,* 2, 56–64.

Karkou, V. and Sanderson, P. (2000) 'Dance movement therapy in UK education.' *Research in Dance Education 1,* 1, 69–85.

Karkou, V. and Sanderson, P. (2001) 'Dance movement therapy in the UK: current orientations of a field emerging from dance education.' *European P.E. Review 7,* 2, 137–155.

Karkou, V. and Sanderson, P. (2006) *Arts Therapies: a Research-Based Map of the Field.* Edinburgh: Elsevier.

Koch, S., Morlinghaus, K. and Fuchs, T. (2007) 'The joy of dance: specific effects of a single dance intervention on psychiatric patients with depression.' *The Arts in Psychotherapy 34,* 340–349.

Laban, R. (1960) *The Mastery of Movement.* London: MacDonald and Evans.

Linesch, D.G. (1988) *Adolescent Art Therapy.* New York: Brunner.

McArdle, P., Moseley, D., Quibell, T., Johnson, R., Allen, A., Hammal, D. and leCouteur, A. (2002) 'School-based indicated prevention: a randomized trial of group therapy.' *Journal of Child Psychology and Psychiatry 43,* 6, 705–712.

McQueen, C. (1975) 'Two controlled experiments in music therapy.' *British Journal of Music Therapy 6,* 2–8.

Murray, L. (1998) 'Research into the social purposes of schooling: personal and social education in secondary schools in England and Wales.' *Pastoral Care 16,* 3, 28–35.

National Qualifications online (2005) 'Personal and Social Education.' Avalable at www.ltscotland.org.uk/nq/subjects/personalandsocialeducation.asp, accessed on 13 October 2005.

Nordoff, P. and Robbins, C, (1971) *Therapy in Music for Handicapped Children.* London: Victor Gollancz.

Office for National Statistics (2004) 'Mental Health: The Health of Children and Young People.' Online. Available at www.statistics.gov.uk/cci/nugget.asp?id=853, accessed on 25 October 2005.

Ofsted Report (2005) *Healthy Minds – Promoting Emotional Health and Well-being in Schools: A Summary of Ofsted Report – HMI 2457.*

Osborne, J. (2003) 'Art and the child with autism: therapy or education?' *Early Child Development and Care 173,* 4, 411–423.

Payne, H. (1992a) 'Shut in, Shut out: Dance Movement Therapy with Children and Adolescents.' In H. Payne (ed.) *Dance Movement Therapy: Theory and Practice.* London: Routledge, 39–80.

Payne, H. (1992b) 'Introduction.' In H. Payne (ed.) *Dance Movement Therapy: Theory and Practice.* London: Routledge, 1–17.

Paternite, C.E. and Johnston, T.C. (2005) 'Rationale and strategies for central involvement of educators in effective school-based mental health programmes.' *Journal of Youth and Adolescence 34,* 1, 41–49.

Porrino, L., Rapoport, J., Behar, D., Sceery, W., Ismond, D. and Bunney, W. (1983) 'A naturalistic assessment of the motor activity of hyperactive boys. I. Comparison with normal controls.' *Archives of General Psychiatry 40,* 681–687.

Qualifications and Curriculum Authority (QCA) (2000) *Personal, Social and Health Education at Key Stages 3 and 4: Initial Guidance for Schools.* London: Qualifications and Curriculum Authority.

Rapoport, J., Donnelly, M., Zametkin, A. and Carrougher, J. (1986) 'Situational hyperactivity in a US clinical setting.' *Journal of Child Psychology and Psychiatry 27*, 639–646.

Riley, S. (1999) *Contemporary Art Therapy with Adolescents.* London: Jessica Kingsley Publishers.

Ritter, M. and Low, K.G. (1996) 'Effects of dance/movement therapy: a meta-analysis.' *The Arts in Psychotherapy 23*, 3, 249–260.

Rowing, L. and Holland, J. (2000) 'Grief and school communities: the impact of social context. A comparison between Australia and England.' *Death Studies 24*, 35–50.

Scottish Executive (SE) (2004) 'The New Mental Health Act: A Short Introduction'. Available at www.scotland.gov.uk/Publications/2004/01/18753/31686, accessed on 03 October 2009.

Sherborne, V. (2001) *Developmental Movement for Children.* London: Worth Publishing.

Stanton-Jones, K. (1992) *An Introduction to Dance Movement Therapy in Psychiatry.* London and New York: Tavistock/Routledge.

Waller, D. (1991) *Becoming a Profession: the History of Art Therapy in Britain 1940–1982.* London and New York: Tavistock/Routledge.

Wells, J., Barlow, J. and Stewart-Brown, S. (2003) 'A systematic review of universal approaches to mental health promotion in schools.' *Health Education 103*, 4, 197–220.

Winnicott, D.W. (1965) *The Maturation Process and the Facilitating Environment.* London: Hogarth Press.

Yalom, I.D. (1970) *The Theory and Practice of Group Psychotherapy.* New York: Basic Books.

Chapter 4

Making Space Inside

The Experience of Dramatherapy within a School-based Student Support Unit

Jo Christensen

INTRODUCTION

Setting the scene

Research suggests that the majority of exclusions of students from secondary school occur after a series of minor incidents, rather than being the result of major, one-off incidents. After exclusion the young person is highly unlikely to return to mainstream education. Figures from the English Department for Education, for example, suggest only 15 per cent of secondary school students attended a mainstream school after permanent exclusion (DfE 1995). In 2000–01 the number of students permanently excluded from schools in England reached 9210 (National Literacy Trust 2004). Students aged 13 and 14 accounted for half of these exclusions. The number of boys outnumbered girls by nearly five to one (National Statistics Office 2003).

Drama teachers, who may play a supportive role for students on the verge of being excluded, often expect to see over 600 students over the course of a week, only glimpsing each child for one hour in a class of approximately 30. It is clear that for students 'on the edge' of the school, this brief experience of drama may not be enough.

For three years I managed a student support unit (SSU) in a community college for students aged 11 to 19. The Community College is a rural secondary school that offers comprehensive education to students of mixed gender and ability. The SSU was established as part of the college's social inclusion policy, in direct response to the government initiative to cut down on the number of permanent exclusions. The age and gender of the SSU clientele was found to reflect the statistics stated above. It was within the rationale of the SSU that dramatherapy as a specific intervention was offered to all students who were referred to the unit. The SSU is a setting within the college that has an intentional therapeutic atmosphere. The unit is limited to four full-time student equivalents. The students in the SSU continue to follow the mainstream curriculum provided by teaching staff in the college, and also have one-to-one support from a teaching assistant. When I was working there, weekly group meetings supported the progress of reintegration. All students initially attended the unit on a full-time basis, and this enabled me to work with individual students using dramatherapy. An example of working with a particular child in this environment will be presented here, while associated findings from a small qualitative study carried out in this unit will be presented and discussed.

LITERATURE REVIEW

Nurture groups, first established by educational psychologist Majorie Boxall, demonstrate a strong link to attachment theory (Bowlby 1988, 1998). Spalding (2000, 2001) builds on the concept of nurture groups with a holistically oriented therapeutic intervention: the 'quiet place', which has a 'therapeutic' room within the school where a number of specific therapies may be offered. Modelling this intervention strategy, the SSU is a defined environment within the school that offers a large room, with an adjacent office space for individual therapy work.

Renwick and Spalding (2002) consider the outcomes of therapeutic intervention based around a short-term (six-week) programme in which the issues of stress and self-esteem are considered. Results indicated that interventions, including play therapy (Oaklander 1988) and story-telling and metaphor work (Mills and Crowley 1986) led to a total increase in positive behaviours in primary-aged children. This study was constructed under conditions similar to my research, as it was also limited to considering the impact of short-term therapeutic intervention on the behaviour of children.

Dramatherapy offers a wealth of techniques that may encourage students to develop a sense of attachment to the school, starting primarily with an attachment to the therapeutic relationship itself. Jennings (1990) discusses three modes of generating play in the developmental play (embodiment–projection–role or *EPR*) model. Activites may be structured to enable the client to move through this framework of developmental play. So, for *embodiment* play, tasks may be offered that are sensory dominated and enable the client to respond through the body. The client may then move on to *projective* play, which includes activities such as story-telling that enable the client the opportunity to respond to the outside world. The progression of this model leads to *role-play*, which promotes subjectivity and symbolism and offers the space for an experimentation of roles. These three areas of play were all incorporated within the sessions that feature in this study.

Furthermore, two specific storytelling methods were used within this particular intervention. The *six-part story-making model* (Lahad 1992) offered a starting point that also provided me with an insight into the resilience of the client. In this model a story is created and the therapist takes on the role of doing any writing that is necessary. Already this establishes a different dynamic to the teacher–student relationship, in that the therapist, rather than the student, is involved with 'writing'. The second storytelling method used is Casson's (2002) *five story structure*. This approach uses a physical, transparent structure that has five open levels, rather like a three-dimensional chess board. The client is encouraged to use small objects/buttons to represent aspects of the self, other people or perhaps characters in a story. There is flexibility in how to use the structure. The sessions featured within this study required the client to choose a button to represent the self and then to consider the self in relation to other family members and friends. Work then considered positive aspects of the self, again representing these through projection onto the objects and buttons. This method encourages the client to represent internal relationships onto an external miniature world, providing an opportunity for deeper understanding of the self.

THE STUDY

Research questions

In the study I completed in the SSU, I wanted to consider how previous experiences of exclusion, or perceptions about the threat of exclusion, impacted upon students, males in particular, who felt it was difficult to belong. As previously stated, according to the National Statistics Office (2001), it is males that account for the majority of exclusions. The question that led my research was: what are the experiences and perceptions of an adolescent boy in a SSU of the contribution that dramatherapy can make regarding reintegration into a community college?

Methodology

In order to move towards an understanding of what this experience might be, a qualitative approach was adopted that followed a case study design. Yin (2003) offers valuable definitions and boundaries for this type of empirical inquiry. A case study enables the researcher to consider contextual conditions (in this case, the SSU) as they are highly relevant to the phenomenon (in this case, experiences of dramatherapy for students who struggle to belong to a secondary school).

All aspects of this research took place within the professional ethics codes of the British Association of Dramatherapists (BADth) and the Health Professions Council (HPC) that is responsible for the state registration of arts therapists. The staff code of conduct of the school was also followed and adhered to issues relevant to child protection. Governors and the headteacher of the school approved the research proposal. Prior to the commencement of the study the issue of recruitment was considered. Consent forms and information about the research and dramatherapy were written, using accessible language, and sent to boys aged 13 who were about to begin a course of dramatherapy. These children were asked if they wanted to participate in the study by a teaching assistant, in order to keep the role of the therapist separate from that of the researcher at the point of recruitment. Selection from this purposeful sample of six was strictly voluntary. The proposed study was discussed between the researcher and each of the children and their guardians. Written permission from guardians was obtained.

Vast amounts of data and observational notes were collected from a wide range of sources. A background of the children, as presented by the children themselves and their school records, informed the process of understanding their current experience of school. For the sake of anonymity the names of the children and their schools were changed. Meetings with external agencies, particularly the educational welfare officer and the child and family social worker, and meetings and telephone-calls with parents or guardians (all of which were logged) were used. Weekly review and target-setting meetings with staff and students, along with weekly record sheets that specifically recorded the progress of reintegration, were also included.

Records from dramatherapy sessions documented the process and the techniques used. The work undertaken in sessions was varied, and numerous techniques were used to elicit themes and to maintain an essential child-centred approach (Rogers 2000). This includes the embodiment–projection–role model established by Jennings (1990), the *six-part story-making model* (Lahad 1992) and the *five-story self structure model* (Casson 2002, 2004a, 2004b). Each of these specific methods was used with each of the participants. Supervision was received separately for the roles of therapist and researcher throughout the research.

Interviews with the children took place after a minimum of six sessions. From these interviews it was possible to develop a case description that emerged from the children's experience, using thematic analysis of the interview as a starting point, rather than a description led by notes and perceptions of the therapist/researcher. It was not viable for these to be carried out by a colleague, as I was the only trained dramatherapist in the school, and as such could listen and follow the descriptions of dramatherapy techniques and process in some depth. The children read sections from the interviews that were to be included in the final report, enabling them to check if their views were expressed accurately.

The case study that will be presented here involves an adolescent boy (I shall call him Tom) who attended dramatherapy in a SSU as a way of supporting his reintegration to mainstream education. Interview material relating to his experiences of dramatherapy will be included throughout. I offer this example in the hope that I can illustrate how the sense of space (an office within the SSU) provided safe boundaries for a student who needed to consider his relationship to himself and to school. Through my work with this one student I feel there are clear descriptions of how dramatherapy may work to support an understanding of the self in relation to others. My decision to refer to this particular boy also stems from the fact that his articulated experiences bear close resemblance to experiences described by other boys.

Findings and discussion

INTRODUCING TOM

Tom was 11 years old, and joined the college as a Year 7 student at the start of the academic year. Tom was described as a child who exhibits behavioural difficulties, but he had no known learning difficulties. Interestingly, he achieved a high score in national standardized diagnostic tests. In assessments set by the National Foundation for Educational Research (NFER), he appeared in the top 14 per cent of his year group in all three tests: nonverbal, numeracy and literacy. Literacy tests also completed by Tom at the end of the research period indicated that Tom's reading age was 13.9 years of age, almost two years above his actual age. Similarly, in the numeracy test used for his age group, he achieved 100 per cent.

Tom's parents separated when Tom was three years old. Tom lives with his mother and visits his father each weekend. He feels he gets on well with both parents. Tom began his secondary school experience with a placement in the SSU, as he had spent three years with Education out of School (EOS), a tutoring provision for students who have been excluded from mainstream education.

When interviewed in preparation for him attending dramatherapy sessions, Tom felt that problems began in nursery school when he experienced difficulties with anger, but he could not remember any specific incidents. His mother, in her interview, agreed that Tom's difficulties started manifesting in nursery. This was after his father had left the family home, and also coincided with Tom's favourite childminder changing employment. Clearly the two instances of separation at a stage when he was beginning to have new experiences may have made this quite a frightening time for Tom. Throughout his early school life he continued to exhibit behaviours that manifested in angry outbursts and anxiety.

Tom attended three different primary schools. He was excluded from his last primary school, where he had experienced increasing difficulties when, aged eight, he behaved violently towards a member of staff. Tom was then placed in a Pupil Referral Unit (PRU). Although he was aware of how challenging his return to mainstream education could be, Tom was pleased to be in the SSU and understood the need to accept the extra support offered to him. Tom made a positive start – so much so that he attended a Year 7 activity holiday for three days. Although he did not stay overnight he cites this, along with leaving EOS, as one of the most important milestones in his school life. Tom's school file contains a number of recorded incidents of aggressive behaviour, both verbal and physical.

Tom claimed that he had no memory at all prior to the age of seven. 'Absolutely nothing. There's nothing there' (Session 1). It was perhaps the trauma of his experiences that had led Tom to disconnect past experiences from conscious awareness. Within the SSU, Tom had been observed on a number of occasions hitting his head very hard, either with his fists or against hard surfaces. In an external agency meeting, Tom explained that he hit himself as a 'punishment' when he perceived that he was not 'getting it right'. This behaviour did not present itself during any dramatherapy sessions, and decreased at school considerably as dramatherapy work progressed.

DRAMATHERAPY SESSIONS

The following material is taken from my clinical notes from Session 4, which incorporated EPR techniques.

> The first 20 minutes of the session was spent using the large boy-puppet, operated by placing both hands inside, creating a variety of different characters. The characters were introduced very quickly – some only had time to say their names – and then were killed off in a variety of gruesome ways. Each new character was introduced as a replacement for the last. After this had occurred over 15 times Tom let the puppet remain on the floor, where it had 'died'. He turned to me and stated: 'You are responsible for all of the deaths and must be punished.' Within the drama I protested my innocence, but to no avail. 'You shall be locked up for a very long time. Move to your cell.' Tom directed me to a plastic chair underneath the window that had vertical slat blinds. I was instructed to 'stay there' while he left the room. I sat. I waited. He did not return. Time passed, 19 minutes. I made the decision to ask Tom to return so that the last part of the session could be spent with him present.
>
> When I went into the room next to the dramatherapy space I was amazed to find Tom reading. I asked him if he would like to return and when he looked up he seemed surprised to see me. 'Of course,' he replied. Back in the dramatherapy room I explained that I thought it would be important for him to know what my experience had been. He listened as I described it:
>
> 'When you first went out of the room I wondered what you were going to do, when you were going to return. I expected you to come back quickly, but you didn't. I waited and waited. I didn't know what to do. I didn't know how I should pass the time. You hadn't left me

> with anything, not even a book to read. It was so difficult just sitting there with nothing. I was on my own. I didn't know how long you would be. It felt really, really lonely and a bit frightening as I didn't know what would happen next. It was all really horrible.'
>
> Throughout this description Tom sat in the chair opposite. As I explained how I had felt his face slowly contorted into a frozen scream. His mouth was wide open and his eyes were almost closed. I let this tableau image sit in silence for a moment. Then I said: 'That's how it was for me, Tom. When you left me on my own and I didn't understand why. That's how I felt.' Tom broke the silent scream and he opened his eyes fully; looking at me directly, he said: 'Yes, that's how it is.' (Therapist's notes, Session 4)

The location of the therapeutic space itself, the office being within the unit, enabled the session to continue and the issues of attachment that arose could therefore be discussed. By addressing the impact of his physical dissociation, the action of leaving the room during this session, Tom was invited to consider the impact his actions might have on others, and in so doing, begin to recognize his own feelings.

It is hardly surprising that Tom's experiences of exclusion from education, prior to his placement in the SSU, had resulted in him having very low self-esteem. Drawing from Jennings (1990), the mask exercise used in Session 5 encourages the participant to create two masks: one mask to illustrate what other people thought of Tom, and the other depicting what he thought of himself. In my clinical notes from Session 5, I wrote:

> The work in this session seemed to have focused upon Tom's perceptions of how he saw himself and how he thought others saw him. It had been evident in the SSU that Tom could be very hard on himself. He violently pushed himself and was quick to comment on any shortcomings he thought he may have. This seemed to conflict with his need to be the cleverest and 'best' student. This was a huge challenge for Tom. I presented Tom with two pieces of card that each had the outline of a face. Tom was then asked to draw how he thought other people may see him. Then, on the next piece, he drew how he thought he was. I asked Tom to give each mask a line to say. Then I held each mask in front of my face and spoke the lines I had been given. Other people said: 'He's ugly and angry.' Tom's mask said: 'I'm ugly, fat, stupid and boring.' We discussed these perceptions and talked about the issues surrounding Tom's image of himself.

> We then moved on to use the *five-story self structure* (Casson 2004a) and Tom used buttons/objects to identify six important people/aspects in his life. He then placed these within the Perspex structure and we discussed his use of the levels. Through this work it became clear that another object was needed to represent Tom's new ability to change situations and to reflect upon his own abilities. Tom identified a screw, naming it 'magic screw'.
>
> Towards the end of the session Tom spontaneously changed his comments, defining himself in more positive ways. Other people said: 'He's a nice person, eager to be friends and a bit shy.' Tom himself said: 'I'm overweight, I'm friendly, I love books, I'm sometimes weak-willed and pessimistic.' Tom had developed a sense of himself that has been built on logical binds and a sense of impending, inevitable failure...
>
> ...After the work using the *five-story self structure*, Tom announced that it was the 'magic screw' that had helped him to change the sentences: 'It helped me to realize that I am not a screw up.' (Therapist's notes, Session 5)

Rather than working rigidly with one specific method, it appeared that using a combination of methods – in this instance the *five-story self structure* and mask work – had enabled Tom to effect a positive change in the perceptions held about himself.

INTERVIEW

By the end of his time with me in dramatherapy, Tom stated that he had enjoyed his first half term at the school and was motivated, hoping to return to as many lessons as soon as he could. For him, the weekly target-setting meetings were very important. This was a chance to reflect on what was going right, as well as to consider what lessons could be added to the timetable. He was an avid reader of fantasy books and spent any spare time in the day reading. Tom did not feel that he had a problem with anger any more, but he observed that the SSU could help him with the transition into mainstream school: 'It's just a different environment, just getting used to the change' (Interview transcript).

Tom expressed the opinion that his experience of individual dramatherapy had enabled him to realize things about himself and others. It is possible that for Tom, being an adolescent young man, projective techniques were particularly useful. For example, through the *five-story self structure* Tom learnt that he was not a 'screw up'. Tom acknowledged that he could be very negative about himself and he found benefit through projective play with objects, as 'It helped to clarify what I thought of other people' (Interview transcript).

Tom found benefit from using art in his therapy sessions. He remarked that both finger-painting and the creation of masks had helped him to realize how he saw himself. The initial assessment task, the *six-part story-making model* (Lahad 1992) was seen as 'pointless' by Tom, although as a therapist I find it a very useful assessment tool (Dent-Brown 1999) that also helps to create a clear introduction to the therapeutic relationship when used in the first session.

Tom was keen to be positive about his experiences with dramatherapy, and he was able to distinguish what aspects of the work had been of most help. Some work with a puppet was seen as being unhelpful. However, he also describes using the same puppet to create a myriad of characters and experiencing this as fun. This led him to recall using costumes and hats to create roles that gave him a sense of 'enjoyment' in the therapy session. At the end of the research period Tom considered the future with optimism and envisaged returning to all of his lessons in time. Tom indicated that he wanted to continue with dramatherapy whilst he reintegrated back into mainstream:

> It's sort of like my navigator. [Dramatic voice:] I'm in a car travelling along the highways of school. [Referring to me:] Navigator. Navigator dramatherapy, which way do I go? (Interview transcript.)

At the start of the academic year Tom was spending all of his time in the SSU. After seven weeks in the SSU and six dramatherapy sessions, he had returned to 40 per cent of his timetable. Tom attended ten lessons of his mainstream curriculum each week, spending the rest of his lessons in the SSU. He was well on the way to reintegrating back into mainstream education successfully.

CONCLUSIONS

In this chapter I have aimed to share the experiences and perceptions of one boy in secondary education who was offered dramatherapy within the SSU of a community college. The results reveal the capacity that this boy had to move towards an understanding of his own life. Although it is difficult to separate the effects of the SSU and the intervention of dramatherapy, the data suggest that dramatherapy assisted the process of partial reintegration into the school in a short space of time. This study is useful for arts therapists who are considering the effectiveness of short-term intervention, as it supports the findings of Renwick and Spalding (2002), illustrating that such a short-term programme was experienced by the participant as positive and helpful.

There is an absence of studies that consider the long-term effects of brief dramatherapy with children and adolescents, and this small qualitative study has not managed to address this gap in the literature. Furthermore, this study focused particularly on the individual perceptions and journey of one boy. It would, therefore, be difficult to generalize findings based on this case study alone.

A high proportion of studies on children and adolescents do not include responses from the children themselves, relying instead on the perceptions of parents, teachers or therapists. The research question outlined in this chapter demanded that the voice of the child be included, as it was central to the theme of the investigation. This is perhaps the study's greatest strength. When working with children and young people, involving them directly in the research process may develop our understanding of what can be done to support their growth.

This study also confirms the assertion by Min (2001) that dramatherapists working in schools benefit from the experience of teaching. An awareness of support systems and the ethos of each individual school may enable therapists to locate the environments within a school that might be the most sympathetic to their aims, working in partnership with units and structures that already exist. In this way dramatherapy can become an accessible intervention that can be used in schools to help to address the growing number of permanent exclusions that has been identified in current national statistics.

Furthermore, the study suggests that previous, unresolved experiences of loss and symptoms of pathological grief can affect students' ability to belong to their school. Future studies with students close to exclusion might focus on the link between loss and the inability to form an attachment to school. It would also be worthwhile to carry out studies of dramatherapy, with the aim of drawing comparisons between different school-based units. If educational establishments value their students, then making space for this work is essential, not just for short-term attendance and academic progress, but for developing skills that will support students beyond school.

ACKNOWLEDGEMENTS

With grateful acknowledgement to John Casson and Kim Dent-Brown for sharing unpublished work.

REFERENCES

Bowlby, J. (1988) *A Secure Base: Clinical Applications of Attachment Theory.* London: Routledge.

Bowlby, J. (1998) *Attachment and Loss.* London: Pimlico.

Casson, J.W. (2002) 'Dramatherapy and psychodrama as psychotherapeutic interventions with people who hear voices (auditory hallucinations).' PhD thesis, Manchester Metropolitan University.

Casson, J. (2004a) *Drama, Psychotherapy and Psychosis: Dramatherapy and Psychodrama with People Who Hear Voices.* Hove, East Sussex: Brunner-Routledge.

Casson, J. (2004b) 'The five-story self structure.' Unpublished draft chapter.

Dent-Brown, K. (1999) 'The six-part story method (6PSM) as an aid in the assessment of personality disorder.' *Journal of the British Association of Dramatherapists 21,* 2, 10–14.

DfE (1995) *Final Report to the Department for Education: National Survey of Local Education Authorities' Provision for Children Who Are Out of School by Reason of Exclusion or Otherwise.* London: HMSO.

Jennings, S. (1990) *Dramatherapy with Families, Groups and Individuals: Waiting in the Wings.* London: Jessica Kingsley Publishers.

Lahad, M. (1992) 'Story-making in assessment method for coping with stress: six-piece story-making and BASIC Ph.' In Jennings, S. (ed.) (1992) *Dramatherapy Theory and Practice II.* London: Routledge.

Mills, J.C. and Crowley, R.J. (1986) *Therapeutic Metaphors for Children and the Child Within.* New York: Brunner/Mazel.

Min, Y. (2001) 'How total learning challenge has approached co-facilitation and groupwork in schools.' *Dramatherapy 1,* 25–28.

National Literacy Trust (2004) Statistics. Available at www.literacytrust.org.uk/Database/stats/keystatistics.html, accessed on 12 May 2004.

National Statistics Office (2003) *Social Trends No. 33.* HMSO Publications.

Oaklander, V. (1988) *Windows to Our Children.* New York: The Gestalt Journal Press.

Renwick, F. and Spalding, B. (2002) '"A quiet place" project: an evaluation of early therapeutic intervention within mainstream schools.' *British Journal of Special Education 29,* 3, 144–149.

Rogers, C.R. (2000) *Client-centered Therapy.* London: Constable.

Spalding, B. (2000) 'The contribution of a "quiet place" to early intervention strategies for children with emotional and behavioural difficulties in mainstream schools.' *British Journal of Special Education 27,* 3, 129–134.

Spalding, B. (2001) 'A quiet place: a healing environment.' *Support for Learning 16,* 2, 69–73.

Yin, R.K. (2003) *Case Study Research: Design and Methods.* London: Sage.

Chapter 5

Solution-focused Brief Dramatherapy Group Work

Working with Children in Mainstream Education in Sri Lanka

Genevieve Smyth

INTRODUCTION

Setting the scene

While working as a dramatherapist in Asia in 2007, I arrived in Colombo, the capital of Sri Lanka, to be welcomed into the city's largest mainstream school. The children I worked with there were 10- to 17-year-olds who had a range of personal and social problems to deal with. These included the impact of urban poverty, the ecological and psychological impact of the 2005 tsunami, and ongoing civil war.

Sri Lankans understood clearly the value of education, personal development and co-operation as the passport to a potentially brighter future. The learning curriculum paid attention to physical and social development through its ambitious sports and arts programmes. In addition, since its inception in 1981, Colombo's Children's Book Society had grown into the largest of its kind in the world for a single country, with 300,000 readers. The Book Society served as an additional education system to support children's mental health development, giving what its president described to me as 'food for the brain'.

The intensive solution-focused brief dramatherapy programme that I delivered during the winter of 2007 was designed to support children's mental health through personal and social development. While I found no evidence of professional training in dramatherapy in the country, in the process of gaining a project award from the British Association of Dramatherapists for this work, I learnt from a university academic in Jaffna that the government wished to see formalized his therapeutic application of traditional dramatic arts with vulnerable young people. The fact that the dramatherapy programme I offered in Colombo was school-based shaped the type of planning required to produce therapeutic results. This was exemplified by the careful structuring of tightly boundaried sessions within the existing curriculum and including staff as therapy translators. Such preparation enabled the delivery of dramatic group work to promote greater mental health.

LITERATURE REVIEW

In my literature review of English publications in the UK and the US, where the profession of dramatherapy was licensed, I observed the lack of explicit references to a solution-focused brief therapy (SFBT) approach. SFBT describes a time-limited intervention which originated in the US and gained recognition in the early 1990s for swift treatment of diverse psychological conditions. While initial work was with adults, the model was later adapted for use with younger, less verbal clients (Selekman 1997). In his article researching clinical effectiveness, Rothwell (2005) described how SFBT quickly 'focuses on clients' strengths and expressed goals in an attempt to produce therapeutic change' (p.402).

On the internet I located nine references to SFBT and dramatherapy co-existing within the same document, but an Athens search uncovered no articles combining these subjects. Broadening the search, I located a number of chapters exploring work with children in *Dramatic Approaches to Brief Therapy*, edited by Gersie (1996). For example, Cattanach (1996) described how dramatherapy and play therapy helped to debrief children from different cultures after trauma. While not dealing directly with trauma, my work would relate to the indirect impact on children's perception of seeing their world damaged by national disaster and warfare. Implicit in their healing process was children's ability to find a new language in play and drama with which to express their concerns; one which could facilitate collaborative working through their own unresolved conflicts. In the same book a Dutch dramatherapist outlined methods for dealing with group conflict. These included maintaining a clear focus, managing tensions and containing the work within the time allocated (Van der Wijk 1996).

For examples of a solution-focused approach to brief therapy with children, I returned to Selekman (1997). He saw the model become more 'therapeutically flexible' (p.13) when arts therapies techniques were applied and supportive adults were included in the process. This encouraged me to consider the benefit of teachers offering translation in sessional work when necessary. However, their availability was limited, so clients required a basic understanding of English. In agreement with the group, translators joined a small group of staff, who had supported the establishment of the programme, to witness highlights of the work in a final 'open' session.

Reflecting on Selekman's approach for the purposes of the Sri Lankan programme, I wondered how dramatherapy might relate theoretically to SFBT. Both were client-centred and notably invested in the client's resilience and motivation for change. Perhaps dramatherapy's unique contribution lay in the different levels of therapeutic applications afforded by play and drama. These had been encapsulated in Jennings' (2003) method of dramatherapy where three different types of play were utilized in the process of therapy – *embodiment, projection and role* (EPR). These play types related to three different levels of intervention: the creative-expressive, the task-orientated and the psychotherapeutic. The value of integrating this multi-level dramatherapy approach with SFBT had yet to be fully recognized for its clinical effectiveness, economical value and ability to capitalize on the client's strengths. Selekman (1997) reflected:

> Resilient children have taught researchers a great deal about how to preserve and cope with growing up in high-stress family and social environments. The children's stories describe a combination of individual, familial, and social factors that had a steeling effect on them and empowered them to overcome adversity… (Selekman 1997, p.212)

Selekman introduced to SFBT the tools of play, improvisation, art and narration to help explore, express, process and resolve problems. He framed these components within a systemic approach that acknowledged developmental theory and embraced co-construction with the child.

Returning to the dramatherapy literature: Selekman's approach linked well with work documented in Jones' (2007) book *Drama as Therapy*. Here Jones clarified core processes underlying brief dramatherapy with school-aged children from different cultures. For example, when dramatherapist Colkett (in Jones 2007) worked with child survivors of the 2005 Sri Lankan tsunami, core processes reflected how the children embodied their tsunami experience and began to assimilate and accommodate it through spontaneous play that was later enacted publicly. As I considered the purpose of a final 'open' session, Colkett (in Jones 2007) explained how dramatherapy provided 'a vehicle for expressing the children's life drama of the tsunami' to their local community (p.160).

Despite the cultural and socio-economic reality in Sri Lanka meaning that some children had less time to play or fewer materials to play with, Jones' (2007) explanation of play and drama core processes affirmed my belief that their role in group therapy could be significant: 'Play content in dramatherapy usually includes play with objects and symbolic toys, projective work with objects in the creation of small worlds, rough-and-tumble play or make-believe or dramatic play involving taking on characters and games' (Jones 2007, p.88).

The role of the therapist (or client/group) as witness was highlighted by dramatherapist Lin from Taiwan when she observed how an adolescent female client used a doll as a projective device to help her explore her body image and express creatively what had previously been conveyed through self-injury (in Jones 2007). In South Africa, dramatherapist Meyer noted how the process of role-play enabled her adolescent clients to create sufficient distance from which to first voice their HIV status to peers during brief therapy (in Jones 2007). This demonstrated how the connection between life and drama is 'intentional and essential to the process of change' (Jones 2007, p.118).

Winn (1994) also illustrated change in relation to the 'life–drama connection' (Jones 2007, p.81) in evaluating eight sessions of brief dramatherapy group work for post-traumatic stress disorder:

> The participants...leave the group and re-establish themselves in their social setting, and their experience of the group means that they have already had an opportunity to be creative, try out new ideas and test whether the recounting of their experience can be borne by others who will be supportive and not judgemental of them... (Winn 1994, p.84)

In *Current Approaches to Drama Therapy* (Lewis and Read Johnson 2000), the first US book to provide a researched-based introduction to the field, brief therapy approaches were indicated in two chapters. However, neither is linked to a SFBT approach. One chapter refers to 'brief drama therapy…(which) entails at least 16 sessions' (Emunah 2000, p.81). The other describes The STOP-GAP Method which resonated with a brief, solution-focused way of working (Laffoon and Diamond 2000). Based on Carl Rogers' person-centred approach, the aim was to encourage safe self-exploration, openness, trust, expression of feelings and insight gain. This approach resonated with me as I planned to offer the Sri Lankan group its first experience of dramatherapy. While the aforementioned core processes described helpful techniques of therapeutic value which could be employed as core ingredients of brief dramatherapy, they did not address sequential therapeutic change.

However, in a 1991 paper on dramatherapy, Read Johnson outlined 'a transformative series of stages' where the client:

- 'expresses the material
- confronts and remembers unhelpful or unresolved issues
- works with them.'

(Read Johnson 1991, p.293)

Here, change in the direction of health could be tracked in terms of the client:

- 'owning the experiences
- actively engaging with them in dramatic form
- resolving and integrating the material.'

(Read Johnson 1991, p.293)

These stages, along with Jones' (2007) core processes referred to earlier, would be a useful benchmark to return to when analysing changes that appeared to take place in the brief dramatherapy programme I delivered. The same stages enabled me to explore significant changes in order of occurrence and to consider further how they emerged and were resolved dramatically.

THE STUDY

Aim

While my work in Colombo was multifaceted and broader than the work detailed here, this chapter focuses on how a solution-focused brief dramatherapy group in Sri Lankan education might work through stages of transformation in conflict resolution, using play and drama co-operatively. Given the children's belief that new learning was the passport to prosperity, dramatic activities were fully engaged with and adapted to meet the cultural norms of the group.

Methodology

I attempted to deal with this using the single case study method, which offered a framework for identifying moments of therapeutic change occurring within the treatment programme. As counsellor-researcher McLeod (1994) explained, 'Case methods are also well suited to describing and making sense of processes of change' (p.104). This approach provided a descriptive analysis and meaning that was, from its perspective on subjective reality, specific to the particular set of circumstances in which dramatherapy took place. My primary concern was to see how this specific group responded to a certain type of dramatherapy programme during a defined period of time in a particular location (Robson 1993).

Methods of data collection involved information gathering from session logs, play-based methods of expression (life-mapping diagrams, social games and group-building exercises), reflective discussion and personal process records which utilized insights gained from my empathetic understanding of the children. Further data was collated from open-ended interviews with staff to gain their perspective of the risks to children's mental health. My approach was process-orientated and holistic, beyond cause–effect sequences. Using elements of a 'multi-method strategy' (Yin 1994, p.45) helped me to gather naturally occurring, emergent and qualitative information within the children's natural environment, and, combined with staff feedback, to create a system for classification of unique and diverse data. The collected data was later examined through thematic analysis that consisted of 'Counting (defined as) categorising data and measuring the frequency of occurrence of the categories' (Robson 1993, p.401).

As a dramatherapist 'practitioner-researcher' (Bell 1999, p.9), I also felt able to 'promote action learning and empowerment' (McLeod 1994, p.101) so that children were actively involved in the change process. This in turn allowed me to identify themes arising and interpret them from a solution-focused brief dramatherapy perspective.

Verbal consent for this research was obtained directly from the headmaster, the president of the Book Society hosting my visit, and my clients. To maintain confidentiality, first name initials only were used to identify specific children, and staff and their work locations in the city were not named.

The dramatherapy programme

The dramatherapy programme was designed as a school-based psychological intervention informed by solution-focused brief therapy principles. Once the programme's brief structure was agreed with the Book Society president and school principal, operations proceeded as follows.

The children and school staff (class teachers in role as translators) engaged with myself on a daily basis for one-and-a-half hours over a three-week period. As a consequence of time in the initial week being dedicated to programme planning and staff's referral of children, combined with my being unable to offer Sessions 6 and 7 due to illness, only six out of the eight planned sessions were delivered. The final session was an open workshop where group members chose to share with their Book Society president, headteacher and translators aspects of personal and social change that they felt had occurred as a result of dramatherapy.

Referral criteria were broad-based, relating to children and adolescents whose impoverished and/or stressed home-life experience and subsequent group behaviour were understood to be risk factors for achieving and sustaining good mental health. Aged between 10 and 17 years of age, they needed to have a basic understanding of English as a second language, with ability to make (minimum) use of a class teacher in the role of translator, and with an interest in using their skills and experiences of play and drama as part of a therapeutic, rather than an educational or recreational, process. The group presented in this chapter comprised nine boys and one girl, all between 12 and 13 years of age and of mixed academic ability.

To establish a robust structure within which to contain therapeutic group work, I devised and contracted with children clear boundaries and goals, along with regular opportunities to review work-in-progress. I endeavoured to construct a clear and professional working relationship with the group, encouraging members to share feelings honestly. Daily staff meetings for briefing and debriefing on the work were scheduled to monitor programme operations, reduce the likelihood of unrealistic expectations and to communicate any welfare concerns. Aims of the brief dramatherapy focused on completing needs assessment and initiating group-building, moving on to expression of significant feelings and conflict resolution. I hoped that this would engender co-operative group work and children's ability to recognize and reflect on therapeutic changes that had occurred during treatment. To support this, a diversity of methods was available to the group. These were exemplified by projective drawing, sculpting and play with objects, together with social games, exercises in relaxation and assertiveness, role-play conveying group culture, and ongoing reflective discussion.

Findings and discussion

At the beginning of the programme staff expressed the following concerns for vulnerable pupils:

- the enduring responsibilities of children as involuntary carers for siblings and parents living in poverty or chronic sickness
- some families' unrealistically high expectations of their children in examinations and sports performance
- the impact of perceived and actual loss as a result of the tsunami and civil war, and unresolved conflicts within family settings.

Similar categories emerged in discussions with teachers about referral criteria, and from the group itself during the first session that identified initial needs. Table 5.1 shows how themes arose from sessions during the children's increasingly collaborative work. All themes emerging from sessions were listed in sequential order of appearance as the group developed.

Table 5.1 also illustrates collated key themes that helped to address the dramatherapy group therapy goals that dealt with conflict resolution and co-operative play. These goals were, in effect, the criteria on which this exploratory case study would be judged successful (Yin 1994, p.29). The second part of my data analysis searched for examples of transformation (therapeutic change) as a result of group play and drama. In addition, I examined how the dramatization of personal material reflected key themes

Table 5.1 Themes emerging from dramatherapy group work

Session	Activity and props	Sequential theme
1	Children project needs onto a relaxation globe ball while other group members observe and listen	Creating better environments
1	Children agree group work rules, which are recorded on a paper 'thinks bubble' (see Figure 5.1)	Rule-making
1	Children use animal glove puppets and create masked characters to express feelings of alienation and integration	Conflict and reconciliation
2	Children play eye contact games and enjoy rule-breaking	Meet and cheat
2	Children tell stories of personal effort to overcome home conflict, using movement and voice, and explore alternative, more satisfying endings	Dealing with family pressure
3	Children activate their sculpt of a cricket team (where the group had created with their bodies a frozen image of the team playing cricket) to rehearse assertive and considerate team playing	Teamwork
4	Children create a handclap to signify a slap and pass it around the circle until someone shouts 'No!' (clap stops)	Finding one's voice
4	Children mark themselves, a helper and an antagonist on a pre-drawn Life Tree (see Figure 5.2). The group body-sculpt the tree; then role-play its character to seek resolution	Conflict resolution
5	Children play 'Bear and the Honey Pot' where one child role-plays the hunter entering the forest (circle) to steal honey from a sleeping bear. This game was renamed: 'Elephant and Ball' for greater cultural relevance, and replayed many times	Assertive leading and following
6	Children present themselves via 'Killer Wink', 'Cricket', 'No!' and 'Elephant and Ball' (last 'open' session)	Self-revelation in group work

and related therapy goals. Therefore, to complete the data analysis, I returned to the two dramatherapy theorists who featured in the literature review, Read Johnson and Jones, and informed the analysis of data collected for this study. Read Johnson's (1991) 'stages of transformation' could be analysed by noting how children took ownership of their unhelpful or unresolved material, demonstrated their active relationship to it in dramatic form, and resolved and integrated the same material in their lives.

Rather than depicting them in stages, Jones (2007) demonstrated the diversity of transformations occurring within the play and drama:

> Life events are transformed into enacted representations of those events. People encountered in everyday life are transformed into roles or characters. Objects are transformed into representations of something, or are transformed by being given significances which are additional to their concrete properties. (Jones 2007, p.120)

In the group work I observed children rehearsing ways in which to integrate new possibilities into their own everyday life experiences beyond therapy. In this process both personal identity and social relationship had the potential to be transformed.

Let us explore in detail dramatherapy sessions where key themes arose from dramatic activity and transformations that followed. Beginning with need assessment in Session 1, the key themes emerged as creating a better environment; rule-making; conflict and reconciliation. These themes linked to Read Johnson's (1991) stages of transformation in a number of ways. To begin with, the children took ownership of their unresolved need for containment in group work by rule-making on a 'Thinks bubble' (see Figure 5.1).

This reflected their need for a new order and sense of social justice, directly appealing to their own capacity for more solution-focused behaviour. Then they demonstrated their active relationship to thoughts of a safer environment to live in through embodiment play where the globe ball was squeezed for stress relief. After this the group disclosed feelings of injustice about their position in their world which they held, symbolically, in the palm of their hands. The children also found solutions to, and integrated, their experience through use of 'fluppets' (animal glove puppets) which were initially in conflict, then calmed by soothing tones. This was followed by other children in masks debating direction towards a better world. The result was an agreement that progress meant working together co-operatively in order to create a more caring environment.

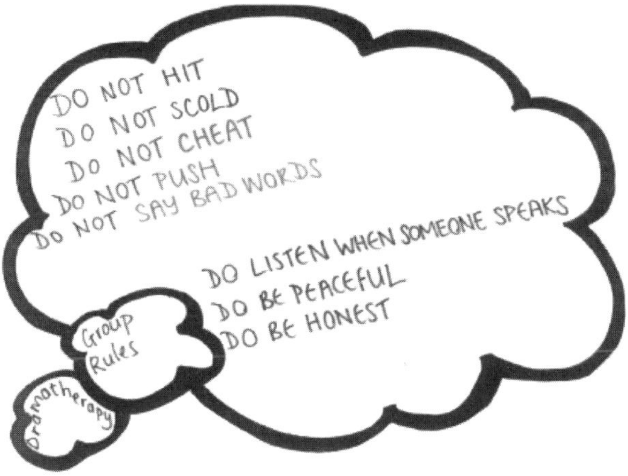
DO NOT HIT
DO NOT SCOLD
DO NOT CHEAT
DO NOT PUSH
DO NOT SAY BAD WORDS
DO LISTEN WHEN SOMEONE SPEAKS
DO BE PEACEFUL
DO BE HONEST
Group Rules
Dramatherapy

Figure 5.1 Group-generated 'thinks bubble' on dramatherapy programme rules

The key themes in Session 1 also related to Jones' dramatic demonstrations of transformation. For example, the life event of rule-making was transformed into a visual representation (see Figure 5.1), which was later enacted and tested through dramatic play. The everyday, real-life characters of group members were changed into masked characters who debated until agreement on a new social strategy. The safe distance created by metaphor enabled the children to speak directly and truthfully for the first time about their experience of conflict at home, where they felt overburdened with family responsibilities. Here the invented dramatic world enabled access and allowed 'explorations which clients might censor or deny in everyday life' (Jones 2007, p.95).

In addition, puppet and mask objects became representations of conflictual relationships until resolution was reached. A third object, the globe for example, was given added value as a device onto which the children could project aspects of themselves or their experience. This enabled each child to gain relief from expressing previously repressed and unsettling feelings, 'and thereby externalize inner conflicts' (Jones 2007, p.84). Having utilized role-play, personification and projection, I witnessed each child achieving a more relaxed state and, in so doing, demonstrating increased capacity for co-operative play. This transformation was identified by children in a reflective discussion where they made connections between the dramas played out and the real lives these dramas represented.

The key theme of Session 3 was teamworking. This was evidenced in children pairing as tropical fruit or jungle animals and in their rehearsing of the cricketing skills of running, aiming, bowling, batting, throwing, catching and observing. Following Read Johnson's (1991) stages of transformation, the children took ownership of unhelpful aspects of their functioning as group members and worked on developing specific life skills, like team playing, with assertion rather than aggression. They engaged with one another actively through creating group sculpts of sporting activities which relied on consistent and fair team playing. Children extended their role repertoire by playing new parts in the game, and later discussed the real-life personal and social benefits of role repertoire expansion.

Session 3's key themes were evident also in links with Jones' transformation theory. This was illustrated as the life event of peer conflict arising from competitive sport became transformed into an enacted representation of the cricket match. Here, moments of unrest could be frozen (to capture and embody the image), rewound and replayed for a more peaceful resolution. Moreover, the everyday real-life characters of group members were changed into the roles of two competing cricket teams. Reflections that followed the de-roling process revealed children's ability and motivation to demonstrate their generosity to other players through their support for the opposition.

Key themes in Session 4 were 'finding one's voice' and conflict resolution. (In role as an antagonist, one child was offered medicine, personal care, love and money.) Related to stages of transformation, each child recognized the need to find her or his own voice by exploring what happened to this voice when the person was treated unfairly. Children then talked of life events when they had lost the courage to speak, and how this comforted the antagonist. The group demonstrated its active relationship to the concept of lost identity by staging a series of 'life trees' which enabled protagonists to examine feelings associated with failure, danger and loss. The group found solution to, and integrated, their experience through discovering their capacity to identify with and name feelings of inadequacy, then to use this to empathize with others, which aided reconciliation.

Links between this session's key themes and Jones' (2007) understanding of transformation were evident in core process work which helped each child to find her or his sense of self in different dramatic ways. The life event of being challenged by an antagonist was transformed into an enacted representation by life-tree work where group members positioned themselves and significant others on a group-sculpted version of the tree (an embodied image; the group members each arrange themselves in a physical position to represent a part of the tree) and dramatized dialogues between characters. These dialogues presented relationship problems in need of resolution. In addition, the everyday real-life characters of group members and family members were changed into the roles of tree dwellers, each reflecting a different relationship to the protagonist group member whose tree it was. While rapport between the protagonist and her or his nominated helper promoted empathy, other characters' identification with the relationship problem generated diverse solutions which were tested out within the enactment. Ultimately the protagonist chose the life-story ending that he or she could best work with in real-life. This enabled child S to self-assess the risk and resilience factors in her real-life situation, and to conclude that the antagonist was more in need of support than she was!

However, S was also supported in that the life event of her feeling uncomfortable in being silent in front of the dramatherapy group was transformed into an enacted life-tree representation. Here the girl used the rules of the drama to give herself the authority she needed to address the group. Changing into a more vocal role paradoxically provided S with sufficient distance to encourage her fuller engagement. Through making the life-drama connection this child retained part of the role to support her active participation in later group work and, uniquely, in home life discussions outside of the dramatherapy space.

Beyond transformations and dramatic enactment, key themes could be linked back to the reviewed literature. Like Colkett's intervention in Sri Lanka (Jones 2007), this dramatherapy programme offered a contained location for stress relief, and support for resolving personal conflict. Here too, experiences were embodied, made sense of and integrated into children's daily lives through co-operative play and semi-structured drama. Reminiscent of Winn's (1994) group work, children seized the opportunity to be playful and enjoyed sharing personal experiences without fear of judgement. This encouraged self-exploration and facilitated insight gain.

In addition, thematic links could be made to the solution-focused brief dramatherapy approach. From assessment to the sharing of group work outcomes, the focus remained on locating children's resources, building on their strengths and maximizing fulfilment of the therapy goals of conflict resolution and co-operative play. This was achieved through the creation of new dramatic languages which could help to express and resolve concerns. Adhering to Van der Wijk's (1996) recommendations, the solution-focused nature of client work enabled me to maintain my focus, manage tensions and contain the work within a brief timescale. Concise target setting, reappraising the past and positively reinforcing the present all contributed to group goals being met. This was illustrated in the final 'open' session where the children demonstrated through selected life-skill games (detailed in Table 5.1, point 6) their ability to co-operate creatively and present collectively some of their life concerns. An appreciative audience commented on the quality of presentation and self-revelation. Overall, the group's commitment to the dramatic process, motivation for change, and ability to realize the transformations, were key factors in the programme's success. In Box 5.1 there is a summary of dramatherapy-related changes that occurred.

Box 5.1: Core processes relating to changes noted by the dramatherapist and child S

1. *Core process: embodiment: dramatizing the body*
   - **Therapist observes**: increased body awareness and confidence in using voice and gestures to express a range of feelings.
   - **Child states**: 'I can say "No!" and put out my hand to stop someone pushing me. Then I feel better.'
2. *Core process: playing*
   - **Therapist observes**: offering and receiving honest feedback.
   - **Child states**: 'I liked your trust game...[in reply] now I trust you.'
3. *Core process: role-playing and personification*
   - **Therapist observes**: recognition and management of feelings of inadequacy and vulnerability.
   - **Child states**: 'When I feel scared, I talk to my doll or draw a picture and then tell my teacher.'
4. *Core process: dramatherapeutic empathy and distancing*
   - **Therapist observes**: capacity to empathize and engaging meaningfully with peers.

- **Child states**: 'I think she is sad in the group today. We can help her play with us.'

5. *Core process: transformation*
    - **Therapist observes**: expansion of role repertoire for psychological and social benefits.
    - **Child states**: 'I am small but now I can play a big person.'

6. *Core process: transformation*
    - **Therapist observes**: conflict management leading to conflict resolution.
    - **Child states**: 'Now I say "sorry" and people like me again.'

7. *Core process: life drama connection*
    - **Therapist observes**: co-operative play.
    - **Child states**: 'It is important to play well with my friends today. They will help me tomorrow.'

CONCLUSIONS

Research findings indicated how Sri Lankan school children utilized responsibly their unique experience of solution-focused brief dramatherapy for the fulfilment of two therapeutic goals: conflict resolution and co-operative play. While brief interventions do not meet all needs, small changes were valued, as one child reflected: 'We can stop the slap being passed around. We turn the other way and it disappears.'

As illustrated in the summary of changes occurring, those experienced in achieving the stated goals appeared to relate back to Jones' (2007) core processes at the heart of dramatherapy. At play within the solution-focused approach to brief dramatherapy that has been presented in this chapter was evidence of both Jones' (2007) and Read Johnson's (1991) theories of transformation. By focusing on the children's responses to play and drama as therapeutic mediums, I believe specific changes came about within a particular time and place in Sri Lanka. This was helped by the extent of the culturally specific creativity and motivation of the research group. These changes were endorsed by an external audience in the final session, and this in itself influenced the change process, in that the group played even more confidently to the new audience. The heightened awareness of both the risks to child mental health, and the resilience factors needing to be nurtured during adolescence, was evident in one teacher's consideration: 'I now see how concerned our children are about their future and how their ability to work together makes things better for all of us.'

If this has been the impact of a single solution-focused brief dramatherapy programme in one school, then there should be considerable potential for transformations through further programmes in more schools. Perhaps this puts an onus on those trained and practising dramatherapy in other countries to collaborate on international partnerships which can research and support such an initiative.

REFERENCES

Bell, J. (1999) *Doing Your Research Project: A Guide for First-time Researchers in Education and Social Science.* Buckingham: Open University Press. (First published in 1987.)

Cattanach, A. (1996) 'The Use of Dramatherapy and Play Therapy to Help De-brief Children after the Trauma of Sexual Abuse.' In A. Gersie (ed.) *Dramatic Approaches to Brief Therapy.* London: Jessica Kingsley Publishers.

Colkett, D. (2007) 'Play and Playing. Research Vignette: Children and the Tsunami.' In P. Jones (2007) *Drama as Therapy: Theory, Practice and Research.* (Second edition.) East Sussex: Routledge.

Emunah, R. (2000) 'The Integrative Five-phase Model of Drama Therapy'. In L. Lewis and D. Read Johnson (eds) *Current Approaches in Drama Therapy.* Springfield, IL: Charles C. Thomas Publishers.

Gersie, A. (ed.) (1996) *Dramatic Approaches to Brief Therapy.* London: Jessica Kingsley Publishers.

Jennings, S. (2003) 'Embodiment, Projection and Role.' *The Prompt,* Autumn, 2003, 10–11.

Jones, P. (2007) *Drama as Therapy: Theory, Practice and Research.* East Sussex: Routledge.

Laffoon, D. and Diamond, S. (2000) 'Hitting the Bull's Eye: the STOP-GAP, Method.' In L. Lewis and D. Read Johnson (eds) *Current Approaches in Drama Therapy.* Springfield, IL: Charles C. Thomas Publishers.

Lewis, L. and Read Johnson, D. (eds) (2000) *Current Approaches in Drama Therapy.* Springfield, IL: Charles C. Thomas Publishers.

Lin, S.L. (2007) 'Research Vignette: Maya'. In P. Jones (2007) *Drama as Therapy: Theory, Practice and Research.* East Sussex: Routledge.

McLeod, J. (1994) *Doing Counselling Research.* London: Sage.

Read Johnson, D. (1991) 'The theory and technique of transformations in drama therapy.' *The Arts in Psychotherapy 23,* 293–306.

Robson, C. (1993) *Real World Research.* Oxford: Blackwell. (First published 1993.)

Rothwell, N. (2005) 'How brief is solution-focused brief therapy? A comparative study.' *Clinical Psychology and Psychotherapy 12,* 5, 402.

Selekman, M. (1997) *Solution-focused Therapy with Children.* London: The Guilford Press.

Van der Wijk, J.-B. (1996) 'Brief Dramatherapy with Adolescents'. In A. Gersie (ed.) *Dramatic Approaches to Brief Therapy*. London: Jessica Kingsley Publishers.

Winn, L. (1994) *Post-traumatic Stress Disorder and Dramatherapy*. London: Jessica Kingsley Publishers.

Yin, R.K. (1994) *Case Study Research: Design and Methods*. London: Sage.

Chapter 6

The Searching Drama of Disaffection

Dramatherapy Groups in a Whole-school Context

Toby Quibell

INTRODUCTION

Setting the scene

A man in a suit sits alone in a circle of chairs, waiting for eight Year 9 (14-year-old) pupils. 'Why is it always Year 9?' he wonders, feeling nervous and uncharitable. The door opens and he gets up to greet the young men and women who crowd the room in all the glory of their ruckus and aftershave. As the session progresses, the youths run through a practised repertoire of hormonally fuelled bonding and conflict behaviours, most of which are fielded by the suited man. He works hard to engage these shambling encyclopaedias of noise and conflict in simple group games, with the aim of establishing a safe therapeutic space. At the end of the session one of the pack leaders begins the feedback. The man leans forward to listen. '...this is all right actually, because at first we thought you were a banker...' The man smiles in a friendly fashion and straightens his tie. He thinks he heard it right...

Schools are places rich with opportunity to make a positive contribution to the development of young people, but given the pressures to raise standards year after year, school life often sidelines the emotional and social aspects of learning. The effect of this is to create a problem population who cannot or will not connect with the taught curriculum – the disaffected. Schools can then get caught up in a spiral of zero-tolerance behaviour management policies that push children towards exclusion. Working with the disaffected in dramatherapy groups engages the emotional and social, and if the work is effective, reduces those anti-social behaviours that inhibit scholastic achievement. Teachers like it when children spend more time on-task in lessons, but the therapeutic methods effective with disaffected children have whole-school implications. How can the school as an institution support the emotional and social development of all pupils? How can the school create an environment where disaffection will be harder to find?

The answer to these questions can be found by identifying effective therapeutic work and applying those elements to the whole-school set-up. If the emotional and social aspects of learning can be effectively addressed through small-group work with disaffected students, these groups could act as exemplars for whole school practice and as a method of shaping a positive, inclusive school ethos. This chapter brings the bruising realities of working with disaffected school children together with published evidence of effective group work practice. I will consider the Action GroupSkills Intervention (AGI) as an example of effective therapeutic group work and ask whether this approach has the potential to be effective in influencing school culture. I conclude by proposing a practical structure for working therapeutically with small groups in school.

LITERATURE REVIEW

Disaffection in schools

For the last quarter of a century at least in the UK, the idea that the behaviour of children is becoming more unruly and uncontrolled has seldom been absent from newspaper reports and political discussion (Batmanghelidjh 2007; Pearson 2007). Concerns about the behaviour of students in schools have featured high on the agenda of everybody involved in education for many years now (Elton 1989). Teachers cite classroom behaviour as the major factor in occupational stress (MacBeath *et al.* 2004; Ofsted 2005), due in part to increased emphasis on raising academic standards and the corresponding decrease in time available for children with attitudes and dispositions that make them disinclined to engage with the curriculum.

Disaffected children are those with unmet social and emotional needs, and despite headline activity in the UK to spotlight this group (Secondary SEAL 2008), there remains some uncertainty as to how to implement practice.

Therapeutic group work appears to offer a good solution to this uncertainty: it can be applied preventatively, it is naturally socializing, it is a good use of resources and it provides a safe space within which sensitive emotional issues can be moved towards resolution. However, when such approaches are systematically researched, they report positive effects that are small, inconsistent and not generally sustained (DiCenso *et al.* 2002; Faggiano *et al.* 2005; Foxcroft *et al.* 2002; Peterson *et al.* 2000; Thomas and Perera 2006). These interventions will work in one school and not in another, with one group and not another, with one person and not someone else. In addition, therapeutic group work is not the same thing as dramatherapy, although certain elements and techniques may feature in both. References to systematically researched dramatherapy in schools are very hard to find, and in the UK are likely to use the Help Starts Here programme as a touchstone (Kolvin *et al.* 1981). For practitioners trying to build up a picture of what makes effective practice, this is puzzling. If an intervention is to stand a good chance of success the next time we want it to work, it should be possible to know what to do to translate it from the last time it was used. When researchers try to control the elements of practice so that the conclusions are transferable and repeatable, they often establish a randomized controlled trial (RCT). RCTs that refer to therapeutic group work are rare, but not unheard of. Together with colleagues in health and education I have been involved in the delivery and research of a programme called the Action GroupSkills Intervention (AGI). This intervention was developed in schools of the Northeast of England as a response to social unease in an inner-city housing estate, in the form of school truancy. The AGI is a dramatherapy intervention, with its emphasis on the creation of a safe space for emotional expression in the form of enacted scenarios. The AGI has published RCT data to support its effectiveness over the short, medium and long term (McArdle *et al.* 2002; McArdle *et al.* 2007; Quibell 2005) – but how can an intervention like the AGI be used to influence whole-school aspects of an 'emotional curriculum'?

Positive school ethos

School ethos can be thought of as institutional culture and, in particular, the extent of student engagement and quality of teacher–student relationships.

What is it that makes one culture different from another? The catchment area of the school can account for some differences in poor behaviour and exclusion rates, illegal drug use and teenage pregnancy, but there are many schools with high-risk populations that have low levels of exclusion (Department for Education and Skills 2004). The schools succeeding in challenging circumstances are those characterized by a school curriculum used to successfully promote protective attitudes and skills relating to (mental) health (Botvin *et al.* 1995; Ellickson and Bell 1990; Ellickson *et al.* 2003). Good practice has also been linked to addressing a range of inter-related issues at the whole school level, in the classroom and in relation to the individual (Botvin *et al.* 1995; Ellickson and Bell 1990; Ellickson *et al.* 2003; Gottfredson, Gottfredson and Hybal 1993; Ofsted 2005; Practitioner's Group on School Behaviour and Discipline 2005). This coincides with advocates of health promotion and school leadership, who argue that addressing organizational processes and social relationships is likely to be effective in bringing about behavioural change (Flay 2000; Moon *et al.* 1999; O'Keefe 1994; World Health Organization/UNESCO/ UNICEF 1992).

Although UK studies have noted that school ethos can add value in terms of examination performance (Stoll, MacBeath and Mortimore 2001), few have explored effects on health and disaffection (Bonell, Fletcher and McCambridge 2007). However, the argument that a positive social milieu can impact on disaffection is supported by a recently published review of the Behaviour Improvement Programme that was developed as part of the UK government's Street Crime Initiative (Hallam 2007). Likewise, high-quality randomized trials in the United States and Australia (Bond *et al.* 2004; Flay *et al.* 2004; Patton *et al.* 2006) not only show that ethos can affect health measures such as teenage pregnancy, but also indicate that these controlled effects can be demonstrated in the school population.

School culture is important in changing behaviours, and as dramatherapists we ask ourselves how we might influence school culture through running our therapeutic groups. There is a recognized relationship between social milieu and collaborative group work (Blatchford, Kutnick and Baines 1999; Christie *et al.* 2004; Topping 2007), and it is reasonable to start to build a coherent basis for intervention by having some clarity on understanding how the child functions and relates socially to peers, to family members and to authority (Warden and Christie 1997). These therapeutic concerns surface in the Gatehouse study (Bond *et al.* 2004) when it speaks of a theoretical base that recognized the importance of healthy attachments and '...identified three priority areas for action: building a sense of security and trust; increasing skills and opportunities for good communication; and building a sense of positive regard through valued participation in aspects of school life' (p.997). There is an emphasis on creating a place of personal safety and valued participation, which is presented as the essential condition for the content relating to specific skills to take hold. This multilevel intervention addressed whole school risk and protective strategies (Bond, Glover and Godfrey 2001; Patton, Bond and Butler 2003). Also provided were teaching resources delivered to 14-year-olds that allowed students to explore a range of common conflict settings and develop healthy responses. *Importantly a school liaison team that supported staff through professional development was given a high priority by the schools involved* (Bond *et al.* 2004, p.998).

These pieces of evidence commend a broadly therapeutic approach as potentially influential in determining and changing existing school ethos. As dramatherapists we are encouraged by this conclusion, and we look into our practice to isolate and emphasize the elements that we know to be effective. To help us do this, I return to the Action GroupSkills Intervention (AGI) and the randomized controlled data that supports it as a dramatherapy programme. Those of us working to engage schools with the transformational possibilities of dramatherapy can have confidence in the research findings supporting its effectiveness. This confidence will be informed by the discussion of important elements that support and, if needed, change school ethos.

THE STUDY

Aims

Within the context of this study we wanted to find out the answers to the following questions.

1. Is the Action GroupSkills Intervention (AGI) effective in reducing disaffection?
2. Is the AGI more effective than other forms of group work?

Research design

The research team looked at the effects of the AGI on the emotional and social profiles of children, by asking teachers, parents and the children themselves to complete a questionnaire at key points in the intervention. In order to provide data of high quality, the research team went to great lengths to standardize the procedures surrounding the therapeutic work with children. A randomized controlled trial (RCT) design was adopted. The following sections tell the story of how the children were selected, how we structured the different types of group work, how we compared the different types of group work, a brief guide to what happened in the group work, and what the results tell us about effectiveness.

Participants

The selection of children is crucial for the success of the groups, but also as a point of dialogue with existing school structures. Children are screened by teachers working closely with pupils, using pragmatic criteria (see Table 6.1) developed to define disaffected pupils, to include a range of concerns. This is necessary in order to avoid homogeneous groups of teacher-selected boys, troublesome in the classroom and selected due to their high visibility. The criteria are presented to teachers to guide pre-group discussions with the AGI facilitator.

Table 6.1: Criteria for inclusion in the AGI programme

Group criteria	The group will be constituted to reflect the range of concerning behaviours in the classroom. All children will satisfy the general criteria, and one or more of the specific criteria, listed below. Care will be taken to balance the group composition when including children with severe symptoms.
General criteria	The group will consist of children whose performance or appearance in school is of concern, or who are performing consistently below their potential.
Conduct criteria	Recurrent incidence of aggression, intimidation of others, off-task, out of seat, bullying, verbal aggression, inappropriate conduct to teaching staff, truanting, temporary exclusion, unconvincing absence, well-meaning but inappropriate boisterousness.
Affective criteria	Recurrent states of mental absence, sadness, victimization, deep shyness, low esteem, low confidence, social exclusion by peers.
Physical criteria	Unkempt appearance, lack of care for physical self, overweight, small for age, having physical characteristic that attracts negative peer attention.
Social criteria	Known major family problems, social isolation, predictable negative behaviour patterns in given contexts.

The AGI is concerned with helping children to recognize destructive patterns in their behaviour and, by reflecting on their roots in social, emotional and behavioural habits, to change these patterns. Selection for AGI sessions is guided by the fact that identified problem behaviours can run as high as 25 per cent and those at risk a further 25 per cent (Meltzer *et al.* 2000; Quibell 2005), so that in troubled schools 50 per cent of the population stands to benefit significantly. By working with these proportions of a class we aim to have the effect of normalizing the intervention within the school 'offer', and to provide a normative group culture within which behaviours can be socialized.

Randomization and control

Using this procedure, 136 children were selected and randomly allocated to one of two intervention conditions: the AGI (consisting of dramatherapy group work) or curriculum studies group (CSG), consisting of small maths and English study. Once running, these groups were identical in every respect apart from the content of the group work conducted.

Measures and analysis

Children's behaviours were assessed through questionnaires that are recognized as valid and reliable instruments to measure internal states and external behaviours (Achenbach 1991a; Achenbach 1991b; Achenbach 1991c; Braken 1992). Data were collected from teachers, parents and children.

The information from these questionnaires was collected at the following data collection points:

- T1: three months prior to intervention
- T2: immediately prior to intervention
- T3: immediately post intervention
- T4: one year post intervention.

At the end of the research process these data told us how children reacted to being in a group T2–T3 (when we considered the AGI together with the CSG), and we compared that with how they reacted to the normal passage of time T1–T2. We then compared the AGI children with the CSG children to see which intervention produced more positive effects. Finally we looked over the time *after* intervention to see if the gains the children made over intervention were sustained. And we asked whether the gains from the CSG or the AGI group lasted longest.

Using a statistical analysis package for the computer (SPSS) we conducted analyses (t-test and analysis of variance (ANOVA) at each stage detailed above. In statistical language, we were looking to see if the differences (variance) within the groups at each stage were greater than the variance between the groups, using p-values of .05 (95% confidence level) and .01 (99% confidence level). We did all this to try and establish the effectiveness of dramatherapy group work in reducing disaffected behaviours in a way that would be persuasive to the scientific community and generalizable to other contexts (McArdle *et al.* 2002; McArdle *et al.* 2007).

Action GroupSkills Intervention (AGI)

The AGI comprised creative-expressive (Jennings 1993) and psychodrama approaches (Moreno and Moreno 1969), including role-play (Bolton and Heathcote 1999), using a range of dramatic techniques either to heighten the experience or to contain it (Emunah 1994). The AGI focused on the inner states of the children, their relationships to school and family. By providing children with the opportunity to reflect on experience, and by legitimizing the process through sustained attention, the AGI was designed to allow children to feel more at ease with their internal and external states. This familiarity disposed them to be more open to the expectations of the socializing environment. The experience of children outside the classroom could affect all aspects of school performance, as school rarely provided the sufficient opportunity to deal with negative experiences in the home or on the street, or to celebrate significant events in the child's life. The intention of the AGI sessions was to make a systematic and thoughtful programme where children could develop the skills of self-expression and then use them to reflect on experience. This broad aim is broken down into session aims in Table 6.2 below.

Children can be anxious about the sessions when they start, and/or fed-up that they are missing another activity – they are often wondering why they have been chosen to participate. Anxiety leads to fight-or-flight behaviours, and if the group looks like a 'naughty' group, then the behaviours will be naughty and conflictual. Getting a contract outlined is a priority (see Week 1 on Table 6.2), but so is establishing the tone of the sessions. A lot of the work during the initial phase of the intervention is therefore about offering a different interaction to what is the norm in school (see Weeks 1–3 on Table 6.2). This is not permission to be laissez-faire, but it is an invitation to be human, with that human curiosity about the lives and welfare of others in the group. This can be achieved through simple games of throw-the-ball and circle talk. It often helps to combine the teacher approach with the openly human: following a stern set of instructions, make a point of laughing at some small joke, or make some self-depreciating comment.

By Weeks 4 and 5 the rapport with the group should have developed to the point where children can be engaged in an activity of self-disclosure, in order to get at the personal narratives. The self-disclosure may be cloaked in metaphor by using, for example, plastic animals given qualities by group members. These animals have then to survive on an island (drawn on a piece of paper), getting what they need, but also responding to their neighbour (how do a tiger and a sheep negotiate boundaries?). Any 'distance' allowed by the metaphor does not diminish the validity of the discussion and its impact on school life. In such work the facilitator is looking for the patterns that identify children as challenging, and it is the aim of any group activity to provide new possible outcomes by modelling change in these behaviours.

Preparation for closure is also important and retains a sense of safety for the group participants (see Weeks 9–11 on Table 6.2).

Findings and discussion

When looking at the behaviours of the children in the study, teachers consistently reported a significant decline of symptoms (i.e. improvement; see Table 6.3).

Teachers reported this improvement happening over the time of the intervention, and significant improvement still present at follow-up one year later. In addition, teachers reported that children receiving the dramatherapy intervention (AGI) showed more improvement than the curriculum studies group (CSG). From the school's point of view, we can have a high level of confidence in saying that children were seen to improve emotionally and behaviourally as a result of receiving dramatherapeutic group work, and that this group work was better than small groups that were not therapeutic.

Teachers gave positive answers to both the research questions posed above. Children and parents did not experience the changes in the

Table 6.2: Grid of planned AGI aims week by week

(All sessions were of one hour duration)

Week 1	**Week 2**	**Week 3**
• introduction to the group • identification of purpose and skills • playful culture • boundaries and contract.	• re-contracting • re-examination of purpose • playful culture • creative-expressive.	• reflection on purpose • personal responses • individual stories • relating purpose to the individual.
Week 4	**Week 5**	**Week 6**
• sharing personal stories • making stories real in group space • possibility of reforming stories • playful culture.	• mini-closure • skills of dramatic enactment • celebration of process • reflection.	• half-term break.
Week 7	**Week 8**	**Week 9**
• boundaries and contract • reinforcement of purpose • re-introduction to culture • attention to completed work.	• dramatic skills • basic enactment of stories • relating enactment to desired skills.	• elaboration of enacted stories • alternative endings • relating to desired skills • begin closure process.
Week 10	**Week 11**	
• acting 'as-if' skills in place • training for transition • continue closure process • reflection.	• celebration of completed work • closure.	

same way. Parents saw improvements at home happening when there was an intervention; indeed, they said that children having dramatherapeutic group work were improving more than those receiving curriculum group work. Parents did not report that these improvements lasted beyond the end of the intervention.

The data tell us that children experienced emotional and behavioural improvement when the groups were happening, and kept reporting this improvement one year later. They did *not* report that dramatherapeutic group work is better than non-therapeutic work.

Teachers gave us the confidence to wonder why the improvements in school over intervention and follow-up, and the superiority of dramatherapeutic group work, were not observed in the same way among children and their parents. Kolvin *et al.* (1981) also reported that parents responding on the Rutter questionnaire score showed no change at either midline or final follow-up for their junior cohort. In contrast, Kolvin's teacher scale showed significant sustained change associated with group therapy. However, in that study, the findings from parent interview did reveal sustained home-based change associated with intervention, for both age groups. Hence, in the current study it may be that the absence of evidence of sustained home-based change is to some extent linked with the sensitivity to change of different techniques of data gathering. For the children, it seems that there is a feel-good factor associated with participation in group work, and it is encouraging that they still identify themselves as improving 12 months after the groups have finished. It is puzzling that teachers are looking at the same children and telling us that those children who were in the dramatherapy group improved more, while the children do not see their behaviours in the same way. Looking at the data in more detail (Quibell 2005) shows that there is change that echoes that seen by the teachers, but it is not at the levels that allow us to show statistical significance. So it seems that the children are less confident about their improvement – something that could be made worse by the change of school that all children experienced between T3 and T4.

Overall, the data from the teachers give us reason to be confident of emotional and behavioural improvements as a result of group work, with dramatherapy the more effective. These data allow us to look at the parent and child reports and look for reasons why the same effects are not observed outside school. We know that behaviour can be very specific to the context in which it happens, and this may be why the improvements

Table 6.3: Is there statistically significant change? Reported by teachers, parents and children (Quibell 2005)

	All children (AGI + CSG)			AGI more than CSG		
	Teachers	*Parents*	*Children*	*Teachers*	*Parents*	*Children*
Over the intervention period (T1–T3)	Yes	Yes	Yes	Yes	Yes	No
Interventions more than waiting list	Yes	Yes	No			
Over follow-up (T4)	Yes	Yes	Yes	Yes	No	No

in problematic behaviours do not appear with such vigour outside school. This conclusion is consistent with the findings of Kolvin *et al.* (1981).

CONCLUSIONS

Through this research study and the linking of therapeutic groups to school ethos, we were looking for answers to the following questions.

1. *Is the AGI effective in reducing disaffection?*

   The analyses summarized above tell us that we need to look at who is telling us it is effective, and over what kind of timespan. Parents do not seem convinced, but both teachers and children provide evidence to persuade us that yes, AGI is effective over the short and long term.

2. *Is the AGI more effective than other forms of group work?*

   Comparing AGI to small-group curriculum studies, it is the parents and teachers that provide evidence that the AGI is the most effective. In addition there is evidence present in school to say that AGI children are still benefiting one year post-intervention. The children themselves do not seem to distinguish between the interventions (see discussion above), but we can say that overall there is strong evidence to show that AGI is more effective than curriculum-based group work.

3. *Do changes in individual behaviour add up to a change in school ethos?*

   The effect on the school ethos can be inferred from the positive findings in relation to behaviour change. As set out in the first section of this chapter, we are looking for effective kinds of group work to act as exemplars for whole-school practice. Certainly the AGI characteristics echo those identified as essential to shaping a positively inclusive ethos (Ellickson *et al.* 2003). The project impacted on whole school health concerns by using a group work approach focused on the importance of healthy attachments and a sense of security and trust – elements at the heart of AGI practice. In answering the above question, however, we would have to say that the establishment of effective group work is an essential first step, but not enough in itself. Good practice has to be allowed to flourish throughout the school if the effect on ethos is to be observed.

I began the chapter by saying that I believe that well run, effective group work can provide an exemplar for the establishment of a therapeutic school ethos. When the school culture begins to reflect the values that we know are essential to the running of effective groups, then the emotional and social needs of children are being accounted for. This is something that happens all too rarely in school, and it has the capacity to positively enrich all members of a school community. With the vision of this possibility before us, we should be confident that as therapeutic practitioners we are uniquely placed in school to make a difference. If we run groups that are effective for the disaffected, we will be creating a ripple that has the potential to affect an institution.

REFERENCES

Achenbach, T. M. (1991a) *Manual for the Child Behaviour Checklist/4–18 and 1991 Profile.* Burlington, VT: University of Vermont Department of Psychiatry.

Achenbach, T.M. (1991b) *Manual for the Teacher Report Form and 1991 Profile.* Burlington, VT: University of Vermont Department of Psychiatry.

Achenbach, T. M. (1991c) *Manual for the Youth Self Report and 1991 Profile.* Burlington, VT: University of Vermont Department of Psychiatry.

Batmanghelidjh, C. 'The real question: why are our children prepared to kill one another?' *The Independent*, 25 August 2007.

Blatchford, P.B., Kutnick, P.K. and Baines, E.B. (1999) 'The nature and use of classroom groups.' End of Award Report to Economic and Social Research Council (ERSC).

Bolton, G. and Heathcote, D. (1999) *So You Want to Use Role-Play?* Stoke on Trent: Trentham Books.

Bond, L., Glover, S. and Godfrey, C. (2001) 'Building capacity for system-level change in schools: lessons from the Gatehouse Project.' *Health Education Behaviour 28*, 368–383.

Bond, L., Patton, G.C., Glover, S., Carlin, J.B., Butler, H., Thomas, L. and Bowes, G. (2004) 'The Gatehouse Project: can a multilevel school intervention affect emotional wellbeing and health risk behaviours?' *Journal of Epidemiology and Community Health 58*, 997–1003.

Bonell, C., Fletcher, A. and McCambridge, J. (2007) 'Improving school ethos may reduce substance misuse and teenage pregnancy.' *British Medical Journal 334*, 614–616.

Botvin, G.J., Baker, E., Dusenbury, L., Botvin, E.M. and Diaz, T. (1995) 'Long-term follow-up results of a randomized drug abuse prevention trial in a white middle-class population.' *Journal of the American Medical Association 273*, 1106–1112.

Braken, B.A. (1992) *Multidimensional Self Concept Scale.* Austin, TX: PRO-ED Inc.

Christie, D.C., Tolmie, A.T., Howe, C.H., Topping, K.T., Thurston, A.T., Jessiman, E.J., Livingston, K.J. and Donaldson, C.D. (2004) 'The impact of collaborative group work in primary classrooms and the effects of class composition in urban and rural schools.' Teaching and Learning Research Programme Annual Conference Papers.

Department for Education and Skills (2004) 'Permanent exclusions from schools and expulsion appeals, England 2002/3.' (Revised.) London: DfES.

DiCenso, A., Guyatt, G., Willan, A. and Griffith, L. (2002) 'Interventions to reduce unintended pregnancies among adolescents: systematic review of randomized controlled trials.' *British Medical Journal 324*, 1426–1434.

Ellickson, P.L. and Bell, R.M. (1990) 'Drug prevention in junior high: a multi-site longitudinal test.' *Science 247*, 1299–1305.

Ellickson, P.L., McCaffrey, D.F., Ghosh-Dastidar, B. and Longshore, D.L. (2003) 'New inroads in preventing adolescent drug use: results from a large-scale trial project ALERT in middle schools.' *American Journal of Public Health 93*, 1299–1305.

Elton, R. (1989) *The Elton Report: Enquiry into Discipline in Schools.* London: HMSO.

Emunah, R. (1994) *Acting for Real: Drama Therapy Process, Technique and Performance.* Levittown: Brunner/Mazel.

Faggiano, F., Vigna-Taglianti, F.D., Versino, E., Zambon, A., Borraccino, A. and Lemma, P. School-based prevention for illegal drugs use. *Cochrane Database of Systematic Reviews* [(2):CD003020]. 2005.

Flay, B. (2000) 'Approaches to substance use prevention utilizing school curriculum plus environmental social change.' *Addict Behaviour 25*, 861–855.

Flay, B., Graumlich, S., Segawa, E., Burns, J.L. and Holliday, M.Y. (2004) 'Effects of two prevention programs on high risk behaviours among African American youth. A randomized trial.' *Archive of Pediatric Adolescent Medicine 158*, 377–384.

Foxcroft, D.R., Ireland, D., Lowe, G. and Breen, R. (2002) 'Primary prevention for alcohol misuse in young people.' *Cochrane Database of Systematic Reviews 3*, no. CD003024.

Gottfredson, D.C., Gottfredson, G.D. and Hybal, L.G. (1993) 'Managing adolescent behaviour: a multi-year multischool study.' *American Educational Research Journal 30*, 179–215.

Hallam, S. (2007) 'Evaluation of behavioural management in schools: a review of the behaviour improvement programme and the role of behaviour and education support teams.' *Child and Adolescent Mental Health 12*, 3, 106–112.

Jennings, S. (1993) *Playtherapy with Children: A Practitioner's Guide.* Oxford: Blackwell.

Kolvin, I., Forbes-Garside, R., Nicol, A.R., Macmillan, A., Wolstenholme, F. and Leitch, I. (1981) *Help Starts Here: The Maladjusted Child in the Ordinary School.* London: Tavistock.

MacBeath, J., Galton, M., Steward, S. and Page, C. (2004) *A Life in Secondary Teaching: Finding Time for Learning.* Cambridge: National Union of Teachers/Cambridge University Press.

McArdle, P., Moseley, D., Quibell, T., Johnston, R., Allen, A., Hammal, D. and Le-Couteur, A. (2002) 'School-based indicated prevention: a randomized trial of group therapy.' *Journal of Child Psychology and Psychiatry 43*, 6, 705–712.

McArdle, P., Quibell, T., Moseley, D., Johnston, R. Allen, A., Hammal, D. and Le-Couteur, A. (2007) 'Indicated prevention in child and adolescent mental health; three-year follow-up.' Submitted to the American Academy of Child and Adolescent Mental Health 2009.

Meltzer, H., Gatward, R., Goodman, R. and Ford, T. (2000) *Mental Health of Children and Adolescents in Great Britain.* London: The Stationery Office.

Moon, A.M., Mullee, M.A., Rogers, L., Thompson, R.L., Speller, V. and Roderick, P. (1999) 'Helping schools become health-promoting enviroments: an evaluation of the Wessex Healthy Schools Award.' *Health Promotion Institute no. 14,* 111-122.

Moreno, J. and Moreno, Z. (1969) *Psychodrama. Volume 3.* Beacon, NY: Beacon House.

O'Keefe, D.J. (1994) *Truancy in English Secondary Schools.* London: HMSO.

Ofsted (2005) *Managing Challenging Behaviour* . London: OFSTED.

Patton, G., Bond, L. and Butler, H. (2003) 'Changing schools, changing health? The design and implementation of the Gatehouse Project.' *Journal of Adolescent Health 28,* 321–329.

Patton, G.C., Bond, L., Carlin, J.B., Thomas, L., Butler, H., Glover, S. Catalano, R. and Bowes, G. (2006) 'Promoting social inclusion in schools: a group randomized trial of effects on student health, risk behaviour and well-being.' *American Journal of Public Health 96,* 9, 1582–1587.

Pearson, A. 'We should take more children away from their parents.' *Daily Mail* 28 August 2007.

Peterson, A.V., Kealey, K.A., Mann, S.L., Marek, P.M. and Sarason, I.G. (2000) 'Hutchinson smoking prevention project: long-term randomized trial in school-based tobacco use prevention – results on smoking.' *Journal of the National Cancer Institute 92,* 1979–1991.

Practitioner's Group on School Behaviour and Discipline (2005) *The Report of the Practitioner's Group on School Behaviour and Discipline.* London: DfES.

Quibell, T. (2005) 'Meeting the Behaviour Challenge: Effective Group Work for Schools.' Unpublished PhD thesis, University of Newcastle.

Secondary SEAL (2008) *Social and Emotional Aspects of Learning for Secondary School (SEAL).* Secondary National Strategy for School Improvement UK.

Stoll, L., MacBeath, J. and Mortimore, P. (2001) 'Where Next for School Effectiveness and School Improvement?' In J. MacBeath and P. Mortimore (eds) *Improving School Effectiveness* Buckingham: Open University Press.

Thomas, R. and Perera, R. (2006) 'School-based programmes for preventing smoking.' *Cochrane Database of Systematic Reviews, 3,* no. CD001293.

Topping, K.T. (2007) 'Group Work: Transition into Secondary', ESRC end of award report RES-000-22-1382. Swindon: ESRC.

Warden, D. and Christie, D.C. (1997) *Teaching Social Behaviour: Classroom Activities to Foster Interpersonal Awareness.* David Fulton, London.

World Health Organization/UNESCO/UNICEF (1992) *Comprehensive School Health Education: Suggested Guidelines for Action.* Geneva.

Chapter 7

Educational Music Therapy

Theoretical Foundations Explored in Time-limited Group Work Projects with Children

Emma Pethybridge and James Robertson

INTRODUCTION

Setting the scene

This chapter will consider the prospective concept of educational music therapy (Robertson 2000) and the implementation of theoretical influences from this model within a practical context, as already situated within the music education system in Scotland; the rationale for these ideas may resonate with developments in other countries.

Since 1999 the structure of the Scottish education system has comprised the 5–14 Curriculum Guidelines, the Standard Grade Certificate of Education (14–16) and the Higher Still National Qualifications (post-16). This latter development has had the effect of allowing students of all needs and abilities to access courses and qualifications that were previously not available to them. In particular, the provision of teaching and learning opportunities defined as Access Levels 1 and 2 has opened up curricular possibilities for students with additional support needs. In the Education (Additional Support for Learning) (Scotland) Act 2004, a young person is defined as having additional support needs when he or she 'is, or is likely to be unable without the provision of additional support to benefit from school education provided or to be provided for the child or young person' (Scottish Parliament 2004, p.2). A further recent educational initiative in

Scotland is the Curriculum for Excellence, which aims to encourage more learning through practical experiences and to help children and young people from 3–18 to become 'successful learners, confident individuals, responsible citizens and effective contributors ready to play a full part in society now and in the future' (Scottish Executive 2006, p.6).

LITERATURE REVIEW

While the overlap between music education and music therapy has been discussed from different international perspectives (Bruscia 1998; Gascho-White 1996; Kemmelmeyer and Probst 1981; Leite 2002; Schalkwijk 1994; Woodward 2000), the general consensus has been that they are related, yet independent, professions. And while commonalities do exist, the emphasis on curricular frameworks, assessment requirements and class sizes inevitably set apart music education from music therapy. Welch, Ockleford and Zimmermann (2001) comment on the provision of music in special education in England, and their findings indicate a dearth of literature specifically concerned with students who have severe and profound learning difficulties.

One exception to this is the concept of 'special educational music therapy' (Goll 1994). Goll presents a theory and methodology specifically applicable to people with severe and profound learning disabilities. In so doing he seeks to bring together the areas of special education and music therapy, claiming that it is an 'adapted rather than a unique and independent framework' (p.62). He is critical of music therapy interventions, which appear to reinforce the notion that the individual person may be qualitatively different or inferior in relation to other people. One might reasonably infer from Goll that there is a greater need for societal frameworks to make the adaptations necessary for all individuals to function equally and more independently within their respective environments.

In 1996 the American Music Therapy Association published a comprehensive volume of papers concerning music therapy within education (Wilson 1996). Issues discussed include models of service delivery (Johnson 1996), in-service training (Heine 1996) and different settings in which music therapy may take place: these include residential (Farnan 1996) and school-based settings (Coleman 1996) and private practice (Griggs-Drane 1996). The context of mainstream schools is also explored (Darrow 1996), and particular reference is made to the consultative approach that a music therapist might adopt with a music teacher. With regard to this latter approach, Chester, *et al.* (1999) planned and implemented a programme-based, consultative music therapy model for public schools in Texas. The aims of this were to allow more students to receive music therapy provision and for teachers themselves to adopt music therapist-generated strategies. It also sought to encourage greater collaboration across the disciplines and, not least, to maximize the time spent by the therapist in the classrooms. Emphasis was placed on each pupil's Individual Education Plan and the combining of the direct service with the consulting service. The authors concluded that the programme was not only a qualitative success but resulted in 'four music therapists...[serving] 55 teachers with 72 classes on 29 campuses containing 424 students' (p.86).

Educational music therapy – a definition

Robertson (2000) sought to differentiate between forms of music therapy according to the needs of the individual concerned. Within a school context, therefore, an educational dimension to music therapy might reasonably be offered. As can be seen in Table 7.1, this is distinct from clinical music therapy in that the potential now exists to guide the student into areas of learning about music as a result of the musical experience acquired through therapeutic interaction. The intervention of educational music therapy is intended for students whose needs are considered mild or moderate. This may be compared to Bruscia's (1998) definition of an augmentative level within didactic practices in which music therapy 'is used to enhance the efforts of other treatment modalities' (p.163). As such it is concerned with helping pupils to contribute to their environment, whereas within a clinical context greater emphasis would be placed on helping the individual to cope with the environment.

Robertson (2006) later suggests that while the music therapist may commence along therapeutic lines and work towards the personal well-being of the student, a time may come when more specific musical objectives will determine the nature of the activities. This should not be perceived as relinquishing therapy for the sake of teaching; rather, through the process of non-directive teaching, or teaching as an outcome of therapeutic encounter, the well-being of the student might be enhanced further through educational objectives. This may necessitate a degree of verbal discussion in order to draw the student's attention to, for example, musical concepts. Thus, there is a shift from what might be termed subconscious learning towards a more conscious awareness of the learning that has taken place. Underpinning this approach is the emphasis upon the student's needs as the determining factor for subsequent aims and tasks.

Table 7.1: A continuum model (Robertson 2000)

Clinical music therapy	Educational music therapy	Music education	Music profession
• surviving →	• subconscious learning →	• conscious learning →	• training
• coping →	• contributing →	• refining →	• working
• functioning →	• growing →	• focusing →	• informing
• reacting →	• responding (aesthetic) →	• responding (artistic) →	• performing
• learning →			

While this should also be observed within traditional forms of music education, greater priority can be afforded to those who may benefit from educational music therapy.

As stated above, educational music therapy is a prospective concept and is respectful of the fact that within the Health Professions Council (UK) separate training pathways for music therapists working exclusively in education are not available. Furthermore, while there are resources available that may assist teachers as they seek to interact musically with students with additional support needs (e.g. Bean and Oldfield 1991; Lloyd 2008; Nordoff and Robbins 1983; Wigram 2004) it would appear that there is a need for more training opportunities for teachers (music and general). Likewise, there is a need for music therapists to be offered training in order to become more cognisant of key principles and practices of music education.

The rationale for Robertson's (2006) investigation was to notice if motivation existed for theoretical interdependence between music therapy and music education. A suggested model for educational music therapy is outlined in Table 7.2. This model is a process, that a teacher might adopt when working with an individual student's musical contributions. The starting point, therefore, is the student's own ideas, which are without influence from the teacher. This requires the teacher to be fully observant rather than interactive in the initial stages of work. The subsequent reflection on this acts as a plan for future – and more collaborative – involvement. The following section represents one way of taking this theoretical discussion into a practical context within the Youth Music Initiative, as promoted by the Scottish Arts Council.

Table 7.2: Educational music therapy: a suggested model (Robertson 2006)

Stage	Process	Action
Raw response	Observation	Noticing
Personal profile	Reflection	Thinking
Musical meaning	Consideration	Planning
Interactive improvisation	Inter-relation	Doing
Refine response	Examination	Confirming

THE STUDY

Research questions

In light of the discussion thus far, it seems reasonable to suggest that the study can be framed within the following research question:

Can the theoretical underpinnings of educational music therapy be deployed within a practical context? If yes, how?

In order to answer the research question, three subsidiary questions emerged that focused on specific aspects of the suggested model for educational music therapy. These were:

1. In what ways might the aims of educational music therapy help individuals to contribute to their environment?
2. How might specific musical objectives help to determine the nature of subsequent activities?
3. What are the particular ways in which subconscious learning from responding to music might be steered into a more conscious awareness?

Background

In February 2005 the Youth Music Initiative team in East Lothian Council Department of Community Services approached the Music Therapy Children's Service, a partnership between East Lothian Council and NHS East Lothian Community Health Partnership (ELCHP) to develop new and innovative, time-limited projects to meet some of the needs of youngsters with less severe additional support needs, and to integrate their professional approach in new and imaginative ways. Previously the music therapy service had been available mainly to children and young people with additional support needs attending one of four core provisions: a child and family centre, a communication and language provision, a primary and also a secondary school provision for children with severe and complex special educational needs.

Evaluation

In this study, five time-limited projects of music therapy group work in two schools took place. These projects were evaluated through the use of a number of different tools: ongoing music therapy work was filmed at regular intervals, and clips were selected to create a training DVD (East

Lothian Council, NHS Lothian and Scottish Arts Council Youth Music Initiative 2007), which also provided a physical artefact to be reviewed. Evaluation data were collected through direct observation, completion of checklists by parents and teachers with regard to children's behaviours before and after each project, interviews with educational staff directly involved in the groups, and open discussion and questionnaires completed by music specialists and instrumental instructors in response to viewing the DVD.

Participants

Each group had between four and six children and lasted for 30–40 minutes each week for up to 20 weeks. Two groups were in a mainstream primary school and three groups were made up from children attending a language and communication provision attached to a mainstream primary school.

The criteria for selection were that the children would benefit from group work aiming to facilitate positive change in the areas of communication and language skills, social/personal development and emotional well-being. Teachers and/or auxiliary staff were invited to participate in the groups for the full duration of the project. A film crew of two adults came into the schools and filmed the sessions at regular intervals, with consent from parents/carers.

Music therapy intervention

The groups adhered to a philosophy of child-led creative music-making, whilst including some directed activities to facilitate turn-taking, joint play and dialoguing, to encourage participation and self-expression within a small group environment.

Findings and discussion

Some of the findings from the study are presented and discussed in relation to the three sub-questions presented on p.134.

IN WHAT WAYS MIGHT THE AIMS OF EDUCATIONAL MUSIC THERAPY HELP INDIVIDUALS TO CONTRIBUTE TO THEIR ENVIRONMENT?

The following description, based primarily on direct observation from the music therapist, highlights how an eight-year-old girl, Catherine,[7] was able to explore contributing to a group of five children from a language and communication provision and how this transferred to other areas including her music education.

Catherine's raw response within early sessions suggested that she did not enjoy playing as a focus of attention in front of the group, particularly in directed activities. However, she would often seek attention from her peers in other ways and would contribute to the group when everyone was playing together. She did not always start and finish with the group. Her personal profile was discussed with the class teacher, and to enable her to participate more fully in the group, individual therapeutic aims were set as follows:

1. increase ability to lead when the focus of attention
2. increase self-confidence at beginnings
3. participate in group beginnings and endings.

Activities were adapted to encourage Catherine to contribute. When taking turns to lead on the cymbal at the front of the group, on her turn the cymbal was moved and placed in front of her chair. As she continued to resist playing, the therapist mirrored each movement she made through musical improvisation on the piano. Catherine showed awareness of the mirroring and began to lead through her movements. She slowly began to play the cymbal, taking more initiative to lead within active instrumental music-making. A further activity was added in which an instrument was passed around the circle quickly, while the therapist played structured music based on a three-chord progression at the piano. In this activity each child had to touch and experience holding the instrument before passing it on. When the therapist stopped, the child holding the instrument was expected to play a solo, accompanied by the therapist on the piano. Catherine began this activity with very brief solos, making little eye contact. As the group progressed she slowly began to lead, particularly starting and stopping and 'surprising' the therapist.

---

7 All names have been changed to respect confidentiality.

Drum duets were introduced to the group supported by a structured play song (Nordoff and Robbins 1968). Catherine appeared to enjoy exploring dialogues with her peers and the class teacher, and the confidence she developed in this activity began to transfer to other dialogues in the group. She became more involved in turn-taking and joint play. She began to use her voice in a more exploratory manner, and her eye contact increased. She began to take less time to join in activities, and the time that she was able to sustain individual attention increased. She began to participate and perform within the group, and opportunities for learning and teaching or refining responses could now be seen to be more accessible to her.

In Catherine's case some of the skills that she was exploring in music therapy were also evident in other areas of her school life during the project. Having developed a routine of standing in one corner of the playground close to the wall, she began to step out into the playground and say 'hello'. She appeared to be engaging a lot more with the other children at playtime, and particularly initiating contact. The music specialist also commented that, following the project, Catherine was taking a much more active role in the class music sessions. Catherine's mother came to the showing of the DVD and commented that she felt that Catherine had really benefited from the music therapy group work input. Checklist responses completed by her mother before and after the project showed increases from 'occasionally' to 'often' in playing appropriately with peers and making decisions/choices; from 'often' to 'always' in involving herself in adult-led activities and using appropriate gestures and/or actions to get the attention of others; from 'sometimes' to 'often' in using language clearly, having an awareness of how others might be feeling, co-ordinating left and right, initiating new behaviours and joining in games with rules led by peers and from 'occasionally' to 'sometimes' in dominating group activities. They also showed decreases from 'always' to 'sometimes' in anxiety and frustration; 'always' to 'often' in expressing her thoughts and emotions and 'often' to 'sometimes' in becoming over-excited, showing aggressiveness, becoming sulky when asked to do things she did not enjoy, appearing confused, having difficulty making friends her own age and deliberately breaking rules.

HOW MIGHT SPECIFIC MUSICAL OBJECTIVES HELP TO DETERMINE THE NATURE OF SUBSEQUENT ACTIVITIES?

The following extracts from direct observations of the music therapy work highlight ways in which therapeutic and musical objectives could be seen to exist within a continuum in a school context.

Therapeutic objectives recorded for a group of five boys (Group 1) included encouraging awareness of others, following a leader, taking turns, and waiting. As the group progressed, additional aims were to increase ownership of the group interaction and musical direction. A structured play song (Nordoff 1977) was used to encourage each child to follow adult-led direction (conducting), to participate, take turns and wait in the song. It appeared challenging for the group, as it had been demonstrated that they preferred to take turns in sequence around the circle. As they became familiar with an adult-led structure, they were able to explore conducting each other within the group. When the production team for the DVD interviewed the class teacher, she commented, 'They've come to learn that they have to actually think for themselves and work out what to do' (Group 1, East Lothian Council *et al.* 2007). As they became engaged in making music and working as a group, they appeared ready for more specific musical objectives to be introduced for exploration in group improvisation.

Another group (Group 4) began to explore improvisation in a more competitive manner, splitting themselves in two halves to engage in 'battle of the bands'. Whilst the group immediately presented a desire to explore musical objectives, it was considered important to maintain a non-judgemental and safe therapeutic environment, so that when motivational levels or group dynamics changed, the therapist was aware primarily of therapeutic rather than musical objectives. Woodward (2000), having trained in both teaching and therapy, views herself as working within a framework of educational music therapy in which the child's needs are of higher importance than curriculum targets. She suggests, 'therapy is more important than the teaching because learning and teaching opportunities arise naturally from the therapy' (p.97).

Responses from instrumental instructors after watching the DVD (questionnaires completed at In-Service, East Lothian, October 2007) reflected the close link between the Youth Music Initiative group work and the skill of ensemble playing: 'very similar to creative work in groups, choice of instruments, decision making, co-operation, listening, etc. Size of groups main difference and time available'. One respondent suggested integration as a next step, 'to possibly integrate ensemble work and work with a larger group as a method of bringing more students together in music'. Another respondent suggested music therapy for an existing music ensemble: 'I would like a one-off session for one of my string groups, run by a music therapist for many reasons.' This comment highlights the need to explore a bi-directional continuum between therapeutic and educational objectives.

WHAT ARE THE PARTICULAR WAYS IN WHICH SUBCONSCIOUS LEARNING FROM RESPONDING TO MUSIC MIGHT BE STEERED INTO A MORE CONSCIOUS AWARENESS?

Nine-year old Jack plays the cymbal at the front of the group. He plays very fast and loud. He is watching, but often drowns out the therapist. She matches his playing with fast and loud playing on the piano at first, moving towards a structure in a 3/4 idiom with a strong beat on each first beat of the bar. This continues to match his continuous playing but challenges the rigidity, with accented beats creating a sense of pulse and structure. Jack indicates awareness of the therapist's playing and begins to add more contrast to his playing. As he changes, the therapist follows his lead, enhancing strong beats led from the cymbal.

For Jack subconscious learning appears to take place through the musical relationship with the therapist. To increase his conscious awareness, the therapist includes other music activities within the group, in which Jack can lead, starting and stopping with his peers. Verbal acknowledgement of the activities is also encouraged. The following extract is from Week 11.

> *Therapist*: We play all together…
>
> *Jack*: Yeah, and then we [pause, he puts the horn to his mouth and blows once] then do that.
>
> *Therapist*: We play all together…
>
> *Jack*: Yeah, and then you play the piano.
>
> *Therapist*: I'll play the piano.
>
> *Jack*: Yeah, and then we'll all, all together play.
>
> *Therapist*: All together play?
>
> *Jack*: Yeah.

> *Therapist*: OK, and then do you want to tell me when to stop?
>
> *Jack*: OK.
>
> *Therapist*: OK, you tell us when to stop playing all together.
>
> *Jack*: OK.
>
> (East Lothian Council *et al.* 2007).

Leite (2002) discusses ways of providing therapy-related skills for teachers and suggests that, in her opinion, the most fruitful form of training is to be found in the experiential dimension.

> It is my experience that teachers who participate in experiential music sessions seem to apprehend in a more accurate way the principles of music therapy, and later produce assignments that reflect a more flexible and psychologically minded approach to children with disabilities. (Leite 2002, p.15)

Leite (2002) believes this is preferable to a more didactic teaching approach, and that the experiences acquired by the educator can then be safely incorporated into his or her own approach to teaching. When interviewed, some teachers present in the groups felt able to build on skills in the classroom, supporting Leite's views and other theories that promote collaboration between special education and music therapy (Goll 1994).

> I think that we automatically build on it, in that we are always encouraging the children to look at each other when they are talking, to listen, to take turns, to wait till somebody's finished – and because Emma's presented it in such a fun way, that's something we can build on. We can refer back to, remember, when we were playing the drums with Emma, that you had to listen and let someone else play, it's the same when you're talking, you've got to listen. (Teacher's comment, Group 2, East Lothian Council *et al.* 2007)

Table 7.3 reflects on how the findings from the practical context could be viewed within the suggested model for educational music therapy. Observations suggested that each group began with the therapist seeking to provide a space within which each child could make a *raw response* to the instruments, therapist and peers. The musical relationships could then be seen to progress through each stage towards refining responses. The column titled *professional resources* has been added to suggest what the study indicated may occur at each stage, in the professions of music therapy, music education and in collaborative practice.

Table 7.3: Findings from the Youth Music Initiative group work within a suggested model.

Stage	Process	Action	Professional resources
Raw response: individual given access to instruments, therapist, peers, in directed and non-directed group and solo activities.	*Observation*: within the session and by audio/video recording; speaking to other adults in the group.	*Noticing*: musical tendencies and music in relationships.	*Therapy*: framework to enable 'safe', child-led exploration.
Personal profile: assessment period of up to six weeks, after which individual profiles discussed with referrer.	*Reflection*: notes on the group/individual process; clinical supervision.	*Thinking*: what can the child do? How does the child relate to instruments, therapist, peers, and contribute to the environment?	*Therapy*: assessment in/through musical relationships. *Education*: relating therapeutic objectives to educational targets.
Musical meaning: musical responses considered within personal profile and group dynamics.	*Consideration*: what is each child and the group expressing?	*Planning*: planning and adapting musical activities to meet the needs of individuals.	*Therapy*: providing a 'safe' environment to explore self-expression and different ways of being in the music.
Interactive improvisation: structured and non-structured activities designed to meet the needs of individuals in the group.	*Inter-relation*: exploring the musical relationship.	*Doing*: group work activities based on personal profiles.	*Therapy*: creative music activities in small groups planned within a therapeutic framework. *Education*: creative activities often in larger groups with less dedicated time.

Table 7.3: Findings from the Youth Music Initiative group work within a suggested model. *cont.*

Stage	Process	Action	Professional resources
Refine response: introducing ideas for exploration and reflection on developing musical and relationship skills.	*Examination*: a move from subconscious to conscious, through musical or verbal formats.	*Conforming*: contributing to educational or additional support for learning targets.	*Therapy*: conscious awareness of relationships with others developed through musical play. *Education*: conscious awareness of, and employment of, musical objectives.

CONCLUSION

Discussion has shown that, within the Youth Music Initiative short-term music therapy group work design, therapeutic objectives are planned in accordance with raw responses and personal profiles to meet the needs of each child. The findings suggest that, once children are contributing to the music-making environment within a school context and taking ownership of their own musical interaction in small groups, they can become more available to address educational objectives, both musical and non-musical. This finding supports the case for a continuum between music therapy and music education.

Through the process of making and reviewing the DVD, important philosophical differences were also highlighted. Observation and the clips selected for the DVD demonstrated that therapeutic objectives are usually child-led, encouraging ownership within a safe, small-group environment. Responses from music specialists and instructors suggested that musical objectives are often closely linked to curriculum targets and delivered, within mainstream education, in larger groups. Within the actual music-based work with children, boundaries between therapeutic and musical objectives could be seen to depend on the professional perspective of the group facilitator and the context when assessing the needs of each child.

It is recognized that this study was based on a group-work design for short-term projects within the context of a national framework promoting participation and engagement in musical activities, and that it was dependent on both the overall context and the orientation of the therapist. Although the DVD provided a physical artefact for review, there was no direct involvement of music education professionals in the planning or development of the group work. It would therefore seem reasonable to suggest that collaboration between existing health and educational professionals should be considered in practice, and that research should continue in order to explore boundaries and develop alternative context-based training pathways that create a bridge and integrate the professions appropriately.

REFERENCES

Bean, J. and Oldfield, A. (1991) *Pied Piper: Musical Activities to Develop Basic Skills.* Cambridge: Cambridge University Press.

Bruscia, K.E. (1998) *Defining Music Therapy.* (Second edition.) Gilsum, NH: Barcelona Publishers.

Chester, K.K., Holmberg, T.K., Lawrence, M.P. and Thurmond, L.L. (1999) 'A programme-based consultative music therapy model for public schools.' *Music Therapy Perspectives 17,* 2, 82–91.

Coleman, K.A. (1996) 'Music Therapy for Learners with Severe Disabilities in a Public School Setting.' In B.L. Wilson (ed.) *Models of Music Therapy Interventions in School Settings: From Institution to Inclusion.* Silver Spring, MD: The American Music Therapy Association, Inc.

Darrow, A. (1996) 'Research on Mainstreaming: Implications for Music Therapists.' In B.L. Wilson (ed.) *Models of Music Therapy Interventions in School Settings: From Institution to Inclusion.* Silver Spring, MD: The American Music Therapy Association, Inc.

East Lothian Council, NHS Lothian and Scottish Arts Council Youth Music Initiative (eds) (2007) *Music Therapy. Working with Groups.* East Lothian: Cormorant Films [DVD].

Farnan, L.A. (1996) 'Music Therapy for Learners with Severe Disabilities in a Residential Setting.' In B.L. Wilson (ed.) *Models of Music Therapy Interventions in School Settings: From Institution to Inclusion.* Silver Spring, MD: The American Music Therapy Association, Inc.

Gascho-White, W. (1996) 'Music therapy and music education: our common ground; our separate paths.' *Canadian Music Educator 38,* 1, 33–5.

Goll, H.H. (1994) *Special Educational Music Therapy with Persons Who Have Severe/Profound Retardation.* Frankfurt am Main: Peter Lang.

Griggs-Drane, E.R. (1996) 'Implications for Contractual Employment and Private Practice.' In B.L. Wilson (ed.) *Models of Music Therapy Interventions in School Settings: From Institution to Inclusion.* Silver Spring, MD: The American Music Therapy Association, Inc.

Heine, C.C. (1996) 'Inservice Training: A Major Key to Successful Integration of Special Needs Children into Music Education Classes.' In B.L. Wilson (ed.) *Models of Music Therapy Interventions in School Settings: From Institution to Inclusion.* Silver Spring, MD: The American Music Therapy Association, Inc.

Johnson, F.L. (1996) 'Models of Service Delivery.' In B.L. Wilson (ed.) *Models of Music Therapy Interventions in School Settings: From Institution to Inclusion.* Silver Spring, MD: The American Music Therapy Association, Inc.

Kemmelmeyer, K.J. and Probst, W. (1981) *Quellentexte zur Pädagogischen Musiktherapie [Original Writings about Educational Music Therapy].* Regensburg: Bosse.

Leite, T. (2002) 'Music therapy for educators: are we informing or training?' Unpublished paper presented at the 10th World Congress of Music Therapy, 2002. Oxford.

Lloyd, P. (2008) *Let's All Listen: Songs for Group Work in Settings that Include Students with Learning Difficulties and Autism.* London: Jessica Kingsley Publishers.

Nordoff, P. (1977) *Folk Songs for Children to Sing and Play.* Bryn Mawr: Theodore Presser Company.

Nordoff, P. and Robbins, C. (1968) *The Second Book of Children's Play Songs.* Bryn Mawr: Theodore Presser Company.

Nordoff, P. and Robbins, C. (1983) *Music Therapy in Special Education.* St Louis, MO: Magnamusic-Baton.

Robertson, J. (2000) 'An educational model for music therapy: the case for a continuum.' *British Journal of Music Therapy 14,* 1, 41–6.

Robertson, J. (2006) 'The concept of educational music therapy: between intuition and implementation.' Unpublished thesis. Milton Keynes: Open University.

Schalkwijk, F. W. (1994) *Music and People with Developmental Disabilities.* London: Jessica Kingsley Publishers.

Scottish Executive (2006) 'A curriculum for excellence: progress and proposals.' Paper from the Curriculum Review Programme Board. Edinburgh: Crown Copyright.

Scottish Parliament (2004) The Education (Additional Support for Learning) (Scotland) Act 2004. Edinburgh: Crown Copyright.

Welch, G., Ockleford, A. and Zimmermann, S. (2001) *Provision of Music in Special Education (PROMISE).* London: IoE University of London and RNIB.

Wigram, T. (2004) *Improvisation – Methods and Techniques for Music Therapy Clinicians, Educators and Students.* London and Philadelphia: Jessica Kingsley Publishers.

Wilson, B.L. (ed.) (1996) *Models of Music Therapy Interventions in School Settings: From Institution to Inclusion.* Silver Spring, MD: The American Music Therapy Association, Inc.

Woodward, S. (2000) 'A response to James Robertson's "An Educational Model for Music Therapy: The Case for a Continuum".' *British Journal of Music Therapy 14,* 2, 94–98.

Chapter 8

Art Therapy in Education for Children with Specific Learning Difficulties Who Have Experienced Stress and/or Trauma

Unnur Ottarsdottir

INTRODUCTION

Setting the scene

Before conducting the present study I worked in a mainstream secondary school as a special educational teacher and simultaneously as an art therapist within the same lesson/session. I inevitably observed the children from two perspectives: the viewpoint of the special education teacher and the psychodynamic perspective of the art therapist. From this second perspective I became aware of the children's underlying conflicts possibly causing their specific learning difficulties. I wondered whether integrating coursework into art therapy would enhance the children's emotional well-being and facilitate their coursework learning. This experience of working in a mainstream school 14 years ago motivated me to conduct research on art therapy in education, where coursework learning was integrated. My research interest involved children with specific learning difficulties who had experienced stress and/or trauma.

This chapter looks at a research study which was carried out in a mainstream secondary school in Iceland. Attention was paid to whether there were, or had been, stressful and/or traumatic event(s) in the children's lives, which had not been mastered, integrated and worked through, that could have affected their emotional well-being and coursework learning. The research focused on the art therapeutic process of making spontaneous artwork, as well as integrating coursework into the art-making in order to enhance emotional well-being and facilitate coursework learning (Ottarsdottir 2005).

In accordance with the Icelandic government policy 'A School for Everyone', most children in Iceland attend mainstream schools, regardless of whether they have emotional or specific learning difficulties (Lög um grunnskóla 17/2008).[8] Special education is offered on individual and group bases in mainstream schools for children who are in need of it due to, for example, specific learning difficulties such as dyslexia or other difficulties with coursework learning.

In this chapter 'coursework' is a term employed for activities undertaken by the children in order to facilitate learning in certain school subjects. 'Integrating coursework' into art therapy is when the artwork made is about, or includes, coursework material such as letters, words, numbers, spelling etc.

LITERATURE REVIEW

Why integrate coursework learning into art therapy?

Art therapy literature, most of which is based on case studies, contains a general assumption that art-making can assist traumatized patients in processing trauma (Aldridge 1998; Appleton 2001; Chilcote 2007; Johnson 1999; Kalmanowitz and Lloyd 1999; Kozlowska and Hanney 2001; Malchiodi 1998; Meyer 1999; O'Brien 2004; Talwar 2007). The art-making is claimed to provide a means of nonverbal expression (Malchiodi 1998; Meyer 1999), increase hope (Appleton 2001; Kozlowska and Hanney 2001) and provide a safe space for processing the feelings of trauma (Stronach-Buschel 1990).

Rubin (1999) also stated that it is easier for many children to use visual modes of communication before talking about the trauma, because the pain is so great that words can neither reach nor explain it. According to

8 The Compulsory School Act 17/2008.

Meyer (1999), spontaneity and creativity are two of the most important aspects of working through trauma, in order to create a new situation out of an old or traumatic one.

Art can be a medium through which traumatic experiences are recollected and processed (Kozlowska and Hanney 2001; Malchiodi 1998). Art-making provides a method for processing and resolving traumatic memories which often are stored as imagery (Appleton 2001). Johnson (1999) also pointed out that: 'Because the encoding of traumatic memories may be via a "photographic", visual process, a visual media may offer a unique means by which these may come to consciousness' (p.106). Pifalo (2007) also stated that 'Because of the visual nature of traumatic memories, an image-based therapy may offer the most efficient means of accessing, processing, and integrating these split-off fragments…' (p.171). A quantitative study conducted by Lyshak-Stelzer, *et al.* (2007) indicated that art therapy reduces post-traumatic stress disorder (PTSD) symptoms.

The limitations of art-making, when working with traumatized patients, are not widely discussed in art therapy literature. In order to explore further the phenomenon of art-making with traumatized patients, the psychoanalytic paper 'Art and trauma' (Laub and Podell 1995), based on case studies and including artwork and written texts from traumatized authors, is worth looking at more closely. In this paper Laub and Podell agreed with the general art therapeutic claim that artwork '…may be the only possible medium for effective representations of trauma' (p.991) and '…it is only through its indirect and dialogic nature that the art of trauma can come close to representing the emptiness at the core of trauma while still offering the survivor the possibility of repossession and restoration' (p.993).

Furthermore, Laub and Podell (1995) claimed that when a patient has experienced trauma, there are two fundamental factors present. First, there is the loss of the internal other, and second, there is emptiness. Artwork can in some cases repair the loss of the internal other, by means of the dialogue with, and expression of, the artwork. As the dialogue continues between the art and the traumatized person, the emptiness may also appear.

Although Laub and Podell (1995) acknowledged the potential of artwork to represent a traumatic experience they also claimed that it had a limit:

> Indeed, it may be that a traumatic experience extends too far beyond the parameters that define normal life circumstances for it to lend

> itself to recall, analysis or reconstruction: anyone crossing these boundaries cannot necessarily return, a fact to which the suicides of many prominent artists who attempted to deal with trauma testify (p.993).

It is possible, as Laub and Podell claimed, that the pain relating to the trauma included in an artwork may become overwhelming if allowed to surface in excessive quantities in too short a period of time. If this takes place, re-traumatizing may occur.

Rankin (2003), in his discussion of a task-oriented approach within art therapy with traumatized patients, claimed that the task-oriented approach provides a sense of control. Although Rankin did not describe any coursework learning tasks, this idea was important to the present research, where an assumption was made that mastering the task can increase the sense of control and decrease the sense of emptiness and helplessness.

The educational therapist Geddes (1999) claimed that learning tasks can serve as a bridge to mastering anxiety. She explained how, when working with an anxiously attached boy who avoided proximity, focusing on a task helped to create a 'learning space' which reduced his anxiety and encouraged self-esteem. This then made it easier for him to forge a relationship.

According to Laub and Podell (1995), there is a dilemma involved in the art-making process in which, on the one hand, there is a request for dialogue and recollection of traumatic memories, and on the other hand, the risk that the emptiness this brings forth can become too overwhelming. As was employed and studied in the present research, this may be solved in part by integrating the logical, cognitive function of coursework learning into art therapy. It is proposed in the present study that when emptiness and helplessness in relation to the trauma become overwhelming, there may be another direction in which to turn, namely that of mastering the coursework learning task while taking the emotional material into account. When a child gains mastery of coursework learning in a therapeutic context, that mastery may, in turn, give a sense of strength that gradually assists him to come to terms with the difficulty of feeling empty and helpless as a result of the trauma. The present research studied the extent to which the processes of both art therapy and coursework learning come together in the art-making, to strengthen each other and assist the child to integrate the traumatic experience and to learn.

Art therapists working in education generally agree that it is important to incorporate art therapy into schools (e.g. Bush 1997; Dalley 1987; Fehlner 1994; Goodall 1991; Grossman 1990; Harvey 1989; Hautala 2005; Henley 1997; Malchiodi 1997; Moriya 2000; Moser 2005; Pleasant-Metcalf and Rosal 1997; Welsby 1998; Wengrower 2001). However, the literature also reports that education and therapy are often incompatible practices (Wallace and Waller 1990; Woddis 1992). As a result, there are only a few art therapists who have incorporated coursework learning into their practice. For example, Henley (1997) integrated art therapy into the educational process in a classroom setting. Moser (2005), an art therapist from Switzerland, described individual art therapy work with a nine-year-old boy in a school, during which essay writing was integrated into the art therapeutic process. However, Moser (2005) did not discuss possible underlying emotional difficulties that may have interfered with the boy's coursework learning. One difference between Henley's (1997) work and the present study's method involves the setting: while in the present study coursework was integrated into individual art therapy, Henley (1997) worked within a classroom setting. Another difference between the present study's method and both Henley's and Moser's approach is in terms of their conceptual framework: while the present study's conceptual framework fell within both art therapy and educational therapy, educational therapy was not included in the other methods. The inclusion of educational therapy in this study meant that a focus was on the relationship between learning and emotional difficulties where specific learning difficulties were observed from a psychodynamic point of view in relation to underlying conflicts (e.g. Beaumont 1991).

THE STUDY

Research questions

The following research questions were posed in order to investigate further integration of coursework learning into art therapy:

1. *In what ways can coursework be integrated into art therapy through art-making?*
2. *How can art therapy be modified in order to facilitate coursework learning and enhance emotional well-being in children with specific learning difficulties who have experienced stress and/or trauma?*

Methodology

The present study was designed as case studies (Yin 2003) of five children from one school in Iceland. The five children, aged 10 to 14, were selected on the basis of information collected from school grades and from interviews with school personnel. Criteria for selection were that children presented specific learning difficulties that appeared to be a consequence of stress and/or trauma.

Qualitative data comprising artwork, case notes and coursework from 123 sessions were collected and analysed. The children's parents were also interviewed in order to gather background information that contributed to the research data.

Grounded theory (Strauss and Corbin 1998), which values the development of new theory, was applied to the analysis of the qualitative data collected from the case studies. Through grounded theory I drew up categories in order to develop an initial theory of the therapeutic method.

In order to evaluate the impact of the therapeutic method, comparisons were made of: artwork, school grades and psychological tests conducted before and after therapy (Wechsler III IQ test for children (Prifitera and Saklofske 1998); the Child Behaviour Checklist (Achenbach 1991); Attention Deficit/Hyperactivity Disorder Rating Scale-IV (AD/HDRS-IV) (Barkley 1990)). Because of the few cases involved, these data were not analysed through inferential statistics; only descriptive statistics was applied. The findings indicated the impact of the therapeutic method, pointing towards further research.

Intervention

There were a variety of ways in which coursework was integrated into art therapy in the study. The degree of the integration varied, from cases in which art therapy dominated to cases in which education dominated, with a wide variety of integrative modes in between. The educational component was adjusted to psychodynamic thinking by the application of educational therapy theory (e.g. Beaumont 1991).

The children were always free to choose how and what to work with in terms of art-making, art materials and/or coursework. In every session the children were given space to discuss freely and work with whatever topic they wanted. The art materials were kept on the table beside them, so they could reach for them and begin to draw spontaneously if desired. Artwork was spontaneously made on many occasions. If assistance was requested with a specific piece of coursework, I sometimes suggested techniques that included integrating coursework into therapy through art-making. In some cases the child spontaneously integrated coursework into drawings.

According to educational therapy an attempt was made to 'tune in' sensitively to what the children needed, in terms of suggestions about when and how they might integrate the coursework (Dover-Councell 1997). The suggestions I made regarding coursework were, on many occasions, based on what the child was and/or had been spontaneously doing or saying. It was always up to the children whether they worked in the way suggested or in another way.

Findings and discussion

INTEGRATING COURSEWORK INTO ART THERAPY

In the study, particular attention was given to the dimension of integration of coursework within art therapy. 'Dimension' is a scalar quality derived from the application of grounded theory. Art therapy and coursework learning are understood as opposite poles on a scale (Figure 8.1).

Art therapy ———————————————— Coursework learning

Figure 8.1: Scale of art therapy and coursework learning

The following images extracted from one of the five case studies provide examples of stages of the integration where the difference in dimension can be observed on the scale demonstrated in Figure 8.1. I will call the child selected John (which is a pseudonym as his real name has been changed). John was 12 years old at the time of therapy.

John had experienced his parents' divorce at the age of 18 months, followed by the illness and loss of his grandparents, to whom he had been close, a few years later. At the time of therapy his father lived in Sweden, and a recurring theme in the therapy was that he missed his father. John worked with those feelings of loss in treatment through spontaneous art-making that included or excluded coursework learning. John's specific learning difficulty related to reading and writing. It was questioned whether non-integrated emotions relating to his father and other losses were in the way of his coursework learning.

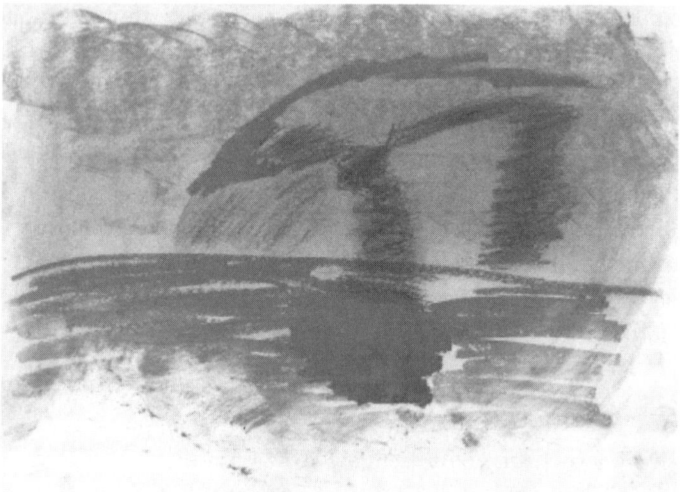

Figure 8.2: Volcano

John drew the image in Figure 8.2 spontaneously, and it had no relation to coursework. This was a volcano that had been erupting for some time. The lava flow could have symbolized John's emotions relating to stress and/or trauma that he had experienced, or feelings of loss for his father and grandparents. According to the theory presented in the study, the expression and processes facilitated by such image-making had the capacity to enable John to process emotions underlying his specific learning difficulties, and thereby facilitated his coursework learning.

The image in Figure 8.3 relates to an example of a move towards a more structured, task-oriented approach, where John had an opportunity to work with his feelings as directly or indirectly as he wished. It was suggested that he drew feelings relating to coursework learning. In this way coursework learning was indirectly introduced into the therapy, which is a move towards the coursework learning end of the scale. John told me that the lower line displayed irritation felt by a boy in his class when reading – which could have been symbolizing his own feelings relating to reading. Those emotions could have been directly related to the incapacity to read fluently, as well as underlying conflicts relating to stress and/or trauma that were in the way of his coursework learning.

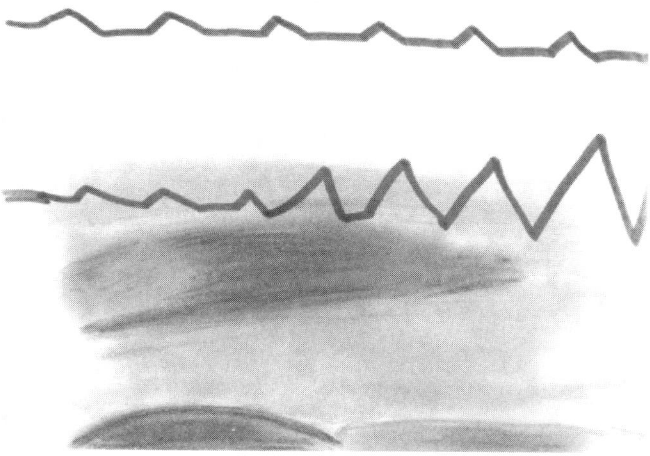

Figure 8.3: Feelings relating to coursework learning

When drawing Figure 8.4, John demonstrated how he had been drawing with his eyes closed at home while he was ill. John continued drawing the same image, adding different, unrelated features, such as his name in a different style, a family tree, somebody reading a fairytale, the sun and earth in the middle of the page looking like a breast, Albert Einstein, Hitler, Stalin, a star and a computer.

As he was drawing, I noticed how fragmented and lacking in coherence the drawing was. Perhaps John was attempting to represent different, fragmented emotions and memories related to stress and/or trauma in order to create a coherent self, comprising different emotional elements represented in his drawings, e.g. his name, the family tree and Hitler. At this stage the task of integration seemed somewhat overwhelming, and his efforts to perform it were disorganized. Similarly, he had difficulties putting letters fluently together in words and sentences that carried a coherent meaning.

John spontaneously integrated words into the imagery in Figure 8.4 without linking it directly to a specific coursework subject. The letters and words do relate to coursework, however, and John's specific learning difficulties had to do with reading and writing. This was a further spontaneous move, therefore, towards the coursework learning end of the scale.

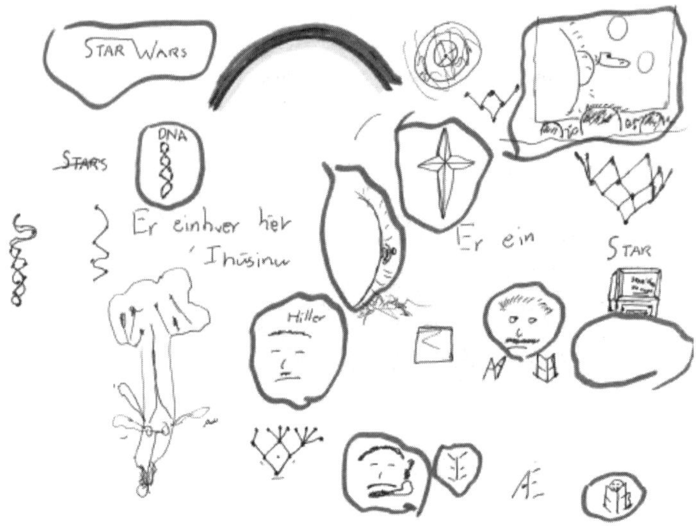

Figure 8.4: Drawing with eyes closed

The starting point of the image in Figure 8.5 was a word that John had written incorrectly in dictation. He had studied a spelling rule about whether to spell a word with 'y' or 'i'. When writing in Icelandic it can be difficult to decide whether to write 'i' or 'y' because the letters sound the same. The word he chose to work with and write correctly this time was 'Tvísýnu' ['uncertainty']. The image is drawn in bright colours and there is a density in the way John filled in the space. There was a view of 'hell' on the left side and 'heaven' on the right side. An art therapeutic interpretation of the image is that he may have been expressing and symbolizing an emotional load, including anger and rage, which he had split off. Simultaneously John worked with coursework in terms of correct spelling (an example is shown in the image in Figure 8.6).

The exercise John completed as shown in the image in Figure 8.6 was closest to coursework on the scale. John practised applying the 'y' spelling rule on which he had worked earlier.

In therapy John went back and forth on the scale of art therapy and coursework learning – as was also the case with the other children participating in the study. The range extended from art therapy to coursework learning with different degrees of integration in between, and the synthesis of both functions occurred in a variety of ways.

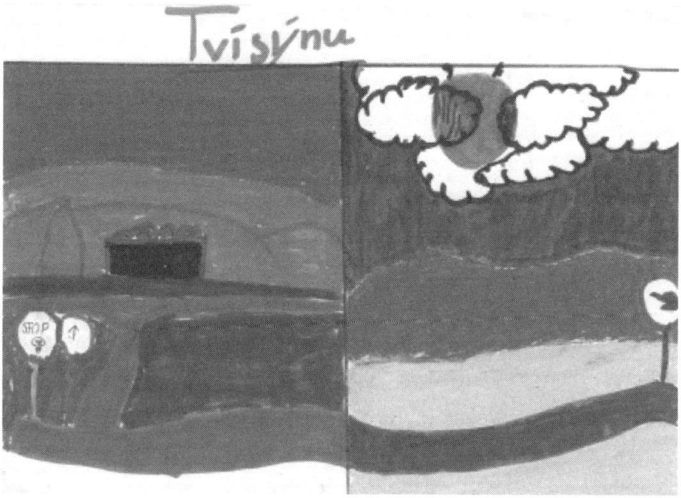

Figure 8.5: Hell and heaven

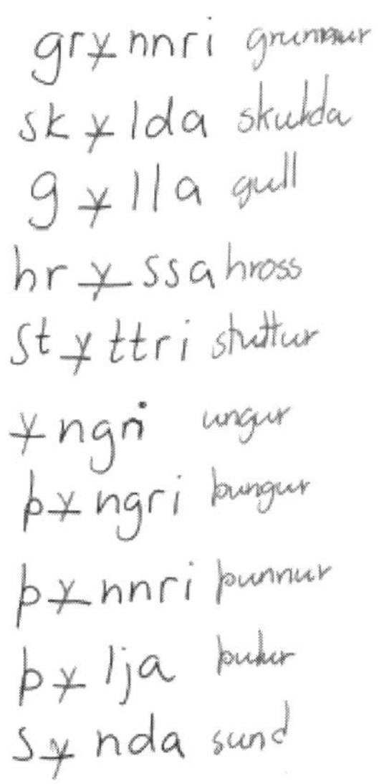

Figure 8.6: The 'y' spelling rule (in Icelandic)

ART EDUCATIONAL THERAPY

The concept of 'art educational therapy' (AET) emerged as the result of the application of grounded theory. AET is the name of the therapeutic method developed through the present study. The theoretical underpinning of AET is grounded in the research data, as well as in the theories of art therapy and educational therapy.

As a result of applying the grounded theory approach, 'integration' emerged as a core category. Dimensions of integrating coursework into art therapy were analysed. The dimensions were manifested in different stages of integration (Figure 8.1). The range was from coursework learning occurring in one session (Figure 8.6) and art therapy in another (Figure 8.2), and between those sessions where coursework learning and art therapy took place simultaneously (Figures 8.3, 8.4 and 8.5). Comparison was made of 1) artwork completed at different stages of therapy 2) school grades before and after therapy 3) psychological testing before and after therapy. Those findings indicated the impact of AET and pointed towards further research.

Findings from the several strands of data indicated that integrating coursework into art therapy can be an effective therapeutic method for children with specific learning difficulties who have experienced stress and/or trauma. Support for this was evident in the comparisons of artwork from different stages of therapy. This included an analysis of developments in areas such as symbolic representation, forms, lines, integration, fullness, lifelines and definition.

The analysis of school grades indicated that the longer the period of therapy, the more positive progress was made in coursework learning. If specific learning difficulties were a symptom of underlying difficulties, and the therapy was of sufficiently long duration, then AET provided an opportunity for the children to work through and integrate emotional difficulties, after which progress in coursework learning followed. This seemed to be the case with John and two other children. Limited or no progress was made in terms of coursework learning for two other boys, possibly because the duration of the therapy was limited and their difficulties were severe.

There was an increase in IQ scores for the three children tested[9] according to the Wechsler III IQ test for children (Prifitera and Saklofske

9 The children were free to choose to conduct the psychological tests or not. Three children completed the Wechsler III IQ test and four did the Child Behaviour Checklist and AD/HDRS-IV.

1998). A significant 16-point increase in IQ scores was found in the case of John. Another boy's IQ score was four points higher after therapy, and one girl's IQ score was seven points higher following therapy.

The results of the Child Behaviour Checklist (Achenbach 1991), rated by the parents, indicated that all the children made progress in some way. John significantly improved his social skills and three other children, each of whom had some symptoms within the clinical range, had no symptoms within the clinical range after therapy. This indicated that the therapy had the potential to enhance the children's emotional well-being, regardless of the duration of therapy. Analysis of the Attention Deficit/Hyperactivity Disorder Rating Scale-IV (AD/HDRS-IV) (Barkley 1990) indicated that, as with the grades, the longer the period of therapy, the more the symptoms decreased.

CONCLUSION

An overarching contribution to knowledge from the present study is designing, studying and testing a therapeutic method of integrating coursework into art therapy, when treating children with specific learning difficulties who have experienced stress and/or trauma. Art-making was found to be a suitable method for integrating coursework into art therapy.

The research project led to the art educational therapeutic (AET) method that successfully enhanced emotional well-being and, when it was of sufficient duration, facilitated coursework learning. At this stage, however, the theory of AET is based on few case studies. It is acknowledged that further study is needed in order to strengthen AET's theoretical base and consider further practical applications.

In AET children have been given an opportunity to approach their memories and emotions relating to stress and/or trauma through both spontaneous drawing and coursework learning. Integrating coursework learning into the art therapy appeared to increase the children's sense of mastery and control and decrease their sense of helplessness and emptiness, which made it easier for them to come to terms with and integrate difficult emotions relating to the stress and/or trauma.

Based on findings from this study, AET is important for several reasons. One is that it is important for children who have experienced stress and/or trauma to have an opportunity to approach some of the emotionally loaded issues through drawing and writing in relation to coursework, in order to acquire strength to work with, and integrate, difficult emotions.

Second, children in AET are able to work with emotional and specific learning difficulties simultaneously. They can work with artistic means within one therapeutic relationship, instead of having to attend two different sessions and form attachments to both an art therapist and a special education teacher. This provides practical and emotional benefits for children.

Third, AET provides children who have experienced stress and/or trauma with a variety of ways to approach and work with their traumatic emotions through artwork and/or coursework. Therefore, it can reach and help children in ways that differ from existing therapeutic interventions, and so additional means to approach the child have been created which potentially makes it possible to reach, work with and help more children.

REFERENCES

Achenbach, T.M. (1991) *Manual for the Child Behaviour Checklist/4–18 and 1991 Profile.* Burlington, VT: University of Vermont, Department of Psychiatry.

Aldridge, F. (1998) 'Images of Trauma in Brief Family Art Therapy.' In D. Sandle (ed.) *Development and Diversity: New Applications in Art Therapy.* London: Free Association Books.

Appleton, V. (2001) 'Avenues of hope: art therapy and the resolution of trauma.' *ARTherapy: Journal of the American Art Therapy Association 18,* 1, 6–13.

Barkley, R.A. (1990) *Attention-Deficit Hyperactivity Disorder: A Handbook for Diagnosis and Treatment.* London: Guilford Press.

Beaumont, M. (1991) 'Reading between the lines: the child's fear of meaning.' *Psychoanalytic Psychotherapy 5,* 2, 261–269.

Bush, J. (1997) *The Handbook of School Art Therapy: Introducing Art Therapy into a School System.* Springfield, IL: Charles C. Thomas Publishers.

Chilcote, R.L. (2007) 'Art therapy with child tsunami survivors in Sri Lanka.' *ARTherapy: Journal of the American Art Therapy Association 24,* 4, 156–162.

Dalley, T. (1987) *Art Therapy and Education. Conference Proceedings.* 'Image and Enactment in Childhood' (pp. 18–23). St Albans: Hertfordshire College of Art and Design.

Dover-Councell, J. (1997) 'Educational therapy.' *Young Minds Bulletin 28,* 12–13.

Fehlner, J.D. (1994) 'Art therapy with learning-blocked, depressed children.' *The Canadian Art Therapy Association Journal 8,* 2, 1–12.

Geddes, H. (1999) 'Attachment behaviour and learning: implications for the pupil, the teacher and the task.' *Educational Therapy and Therapeutic Teaching,* April, 8, 20–34.

Goodall, P. (1991) 'Role Boundaries: Art Therapist or Teacher?' *Art Therapy in Education: The British Association of Art Therapists,* 9–11. From the Annual General Meeting of the British Association of Art Therapists, 6 May 1989.

Grossman, G.S. (1990) 'Spontaneous art: its role in education.' *The Canadian Art Therapy Association Journal 5,* 2, 18–27.

Harvey, S. (1989) 'Creative arts therapies in the classroom: a study of cognitive, emotional, and motivational changes.' *American Journal of Dance Therapy 11,* 2, 85–10.

Hautala, P. (2005) 'Art-therapeutic education as the new way to teach adolescents with learning difficulties.' In L. Kossolapow, S. Scoble and D. Waller (eds) *European Arts Therapy: Different Approaches to a Unique Discipline Opening Regional Portals.* New Brunswick, NJ: Transaction Publishers.

Henley, D. (1997) 'Expressive arts therapy as alternative education: devising a therapeutic curriculum.' *ARTherapy: Journal of the American Art Therapy Association 14,* 1, 15–22.

Johnson, D.R. (1999) *Essays on the Creative Arts Therapies: Imaging the Birth of a Profession.* Springfield, IL: Charles C. Thomas.

Kalmanowitz, D. and Lloyd, B. (1999) 'Fragments of art at work: art therapy in the former Yugoslavia.' *The Arts in Psychotherapy 26,* 1, 15–25.

Kozlowska, K. and Hanney, L. (2001) 'An art therapy group for children traumatized by parental violence and separation.' *Clinical Child Psychology and Psychiatry 6,* 1, 49–78.

Laub, D. and Podell, D. (1995) 'Art and trauma.' *International Journal of Psychoanalysis 76,* 5, 991–1005.

Lyshak-Stelzer, F., Singer, P., John, P.S. and Chemtob, C.M. (2007) 'Art therapy for adolescents with posttraumatic stress disorder symptoms: a pilot study.' *ARTherapy: Journal of the American Art Therapy Association 24,* 4, 163–169.

Lög um grunnskóla (2008) 17/2008. Available at www.menntamalaraduneyti.is/log-og-reglugerdir/, accessed on 6 July 2008.

Malchiodi, C.A. (1997) 'Art therapy in schools.' *ARTherapy: Journal of the American Art Therapy Association 14,* 1, 2–4.

Malchiodi, C.A. (1998) *Understanding Children's Drawings.* London: Jessica Kingsley Publishers.

Meyer, M.A. (1999) 'In Exile from the Body: Creating a "Play Room" in the "Waiting Room".' In S.K. Levine and E.G. Levine (eds) *Foundations of Expressive Art Therapy: Theoretical and Clinical Perspectives.* London: Jessica Kingsley Publishers.

Moriya, D. (2000) *Art Therapy in Schools: Effective Integration of Art Therapists in Schools.* Israel: Dafna Moriya.

Moser, P. (2005) 'Cow-Shed and Vocabulary or: How to Improve Verbal and Interactive Competencies in Art Therapy.' In L. Kossolapow, S. Scoble and D. Waller (eds), *European Arts Therapy: Different Approaches to a Unique Discipline Opening Regional Portals.* New Brunswick, NJ: Transaction Publishers.

O'Brien, F. (2004) 'The making of mess in art therapy: attachment, trauma and the brain.' *Inscape 9,* 1, 2–13.

Ottarsdottir, U. (2005) 'Art therapy in education: for children with specific learning difficulties who have experienced stress and/or trauma.' Unpublished PhD thesis, University of Hertfordshire, Hatfield.

Pifalo, T. (2007) 'Jogging the cogs: trauma-focused art therapy and cognitive behavioural therapy with sexually abused children.' *Art Therapy: Journal of the American Art Therapy Association 24,* 4, 170–175.

Pleasant-Metcalf, A.M. and Rosal, M.L. (1997) 'The use of art therapy to improve academic performance.' *ARTherapy: Journal of the American Art Therapy Association 14,* 1, 23–28.

Prifitera, A. and Saklofske, D. (eds). (1998) *WISC-III: Clinical Use and Interpretation. Scientist–Practitioner Perspectives.* London: Academic Press.

Rankin, A.B. (2003) 'A task-oriented approach to art therapy in trauma treatment.' *ARTherapy: Journal of the American Art Therapy Association 20,* 3, 138–147.

Rubin, J.A. (1999) *Art Therapy: An Introduction.* Philadelphia, PA: Brunner/Mazel.

Stronach-Buschel, B. (1990) 'Trauma, children, and art.' *American Journal of Art Therapy 29,* 11, 48–52.

Strauss, A. and Corbin, J. (1998) *Basics of Qualitative Research: Techniques and Procedures for Developing Grounded Theory.* London: Sage Publications.

Talwar, S. (2007) 'Accessing traumatic memory through art-making: an art therapy trauma protocol (ATTP).' *The Arts in Psychotherapy 34*, 1, 22–35.

Wallace, J. and Waller, D. (1990) 'Art Therapy and Special Education.' In N. Jones (ed.) *Special Educational Needs Review (Vol. 3)*. Sussex: The Falmer Press.

Welsby, C. (1998) 'A part of the whole: art therapy in a girls' comprehensive school.' *Inscape 3*, 1, 33–40.

Wengrower, H. (2001) 'Arts therapies in educational settings: an intercultural encounter.' *The Arts in Psychotherapy 28*, 2, 109–115.

Woddis, J. (1992) 'Art therapy: new problems, new solutions?' In D. Waller and A. Gilroy (eds) *Art Therapy: A Handbook*. Buckingham: Open University Press.

Yin, R.K. (2003) *Case Study Research: Design and Methods*. (Third edition.) London: Sage Publications.

Chapter 9

'Give Me Some Paper'

The Role of Image-making as a Stabilizing Force for a Child in Transition

Frances Prokofiev

INTRODUCTION

Setting the scene

For 13 years I worked as an art therapist in a mainstream primary school with children between the ages of 4 and 11 years. A significant number of my referrals were looked-after children, often in short-term placements waiting for long-term foster parents to be found. They were referred for acute anxiety and sometimes challenging behaviour, which was an 'acting out' of feelings that were barely manageable. The primary goal was to support them through a period of chronic uncertainty, rather than promoting change through the insights gained during the art process. Usually this work would continue until a long-term placement was found and they moved away to their new family and new school.

LITERATURE REVIEW

Looked-after children have usually experienced early life as traumatic. Abuse or neglect often lies behind their removal from their family, so they are likely to have insecure attachments of the most incapacitating kind (Bowlby 1988), which lead to a lack of strategies to cope with stress and an inability to regulate their feelings (Schore 1994). Such children's ability to manage the uncertainty and emotional strain of changes in their home circumstances is therefore dramatically less than that of a child with a secure early life who has developed more mature defences to handle change.

The situation is changing, but it has been the case that looked-after children are not offered therapy until they are established in a permanent home setting which is seen as providing the necessary security for it to begin. While it may be true that making interpretations to a child in emotional pain could feel, as Hoxter (1983, p.130) has said, like 'a cruel stab at an open wound', this is one of the reasons why the arts therapies could be considered ideal in a therapeutic situation where delving deeply should be avoided and supportive therapy be offered to strengthen the ego at a time of threat. When art-making is the focus of therapy, children can feel more control over how the session proceeds. Increasingly the art therapy literature has examples of successful work with children with insecure attachment patterns of behaviour where the emphasis is largely on the containing power of the art process and the calm, containing presence of the art therapist, both of which appear to help the regulation of feelings (Aldridge 1998; Case 2008; O'Brien 2008). Meaning can remain in the metaphor of the picture rather than being interpreted. Without a therapeutic intervention to provide emotional support, it is hard to see how the experience of waiting fearfully and coping with transition can pass without the child suffering more trauma.

THE STUDY

Aim and research question

The purpose of this chapter is to describe part of my ongoing qualitative research into a retrospective single case study. The case consists of four years' art therapy with a White British boy between the ages of four and eight years, starting from his entry into primary school and following him through changes of foster care. I will call him Alistair to preserve anonymity. The research element I focus on here is my research into his artwork using a visual methodology.

My choice of this case for research was influenced by Alistair's enormous output of work (over 600 pictures on paper), the urgency with which he made it (his need for the process), and the apparent success of art therapy in the sense that Alistair could hold himself together sufficiently for some growth to be possible and to access the National Curriculum. In the research reported in this chapter, I seek to understand how image-making helped Alistair contain his feelings at a time of great stress, and what my findings show about the relevance of art therapy as an appropriate intervention for similar looked-after children in transition. So the research question I will address is:

What is the function and meaning of image-making as a containing force in Alistair's art therapy?

Because of the retrospective nature of the work, I will begin by summarizing the narrative of the case study to explain the context in which the pictures were made, and then go on to describe methodological considerations and preliminary findings.

Introducing Alistair

When Alistair arrived at school, aged four, he was a confused boy with no understanding of himself as a member of his class group, or of the world and its meanings. He misread other people's behaviour towards him and was reported by an educational psychologist to have a short attention span, poor fine motor control and behaviour that put him at risk of harm; he had no sense of safe boundaries.

Alistair was the younger of two brothers by 13 months. Although his mother loved her boys, she had a deprived background herself and a history of alcohol and drug abuse, and was barely able to support their needs. She was a victim of a violent marriage and, although her husband left when Alistair was six weeks old, his legacy was embedded in the aggression of Alistair's brother, whose own violence was often directed at Alistair. In school, although Alistair could be aggressive and stubborn, he enchanted adults with his naive questions and many people longed to rescue him. Alistair was referred to art therapy for help with setting boundaries, managing his feelings and developing his understanding of his world.

Nine months into art therapy, Alistair and his brother ran away from home when they found their mother unconscious from drink. They were removed from her care and placed in a hostel for looked-after children while plans were made for their future. This period became two years for Alistair, during which a court decision was made for both boys to be separately placed in long-term foster placements and not to return to their mother. Art therapy became a twice-weekly intervention for most of this middle period. Alistair aroused concern in his early days in the hostel, with his feelings of worthlessness and attempts at self-harm. In particularly stressful periods he regressed to soiling, symbolizing the incontinence of his feelings.

When a long-term foster family was at last found, Alistair moved to a new school and social services asked me to continue art therapy there, to help him with the transition. Now his preoccupations were with the unfamiliarity of his new family's ways and values, worries about his absent brother and mother (whose futures were both unresolved), coupled with anger at having two mothers and the difficulty this contributed to settling down. He was also adjusting to having a father at home and the oedipal feelings this aroused. Most urgently he was worried about whether the new family might reject him if he were not very good.

Methods of data collection

My data for studying Alistair's art therapy included his artwork, my process notes and the reports and review papers from different professionals involved, which included school special needs plans and reviews and teachers' reports, as well as documented conversations between us. The latter material is what confirmed development and progress in Alistair's life outside art therapy.

Methodology

Schaverien (1991) introduced the retrospective review as a research method to investigate meaning in artwork produced in art therapy. This is a development from a 'review session' where art therapist and patient look back through all the art made together, pondering links between works and observing the process with the benefit of hindsight. The expectation is to reach a deeper understanding of the process and images (Schaverien 1995). Gilroy (2006) picks out four stages in this process: a systematic analysis of the physical components of the images; documentation of changes in the images; cross-referencing with the process notes, and comparing patient's and art therapist's experiences where possible.

As there was so much artwork, the only practical way to review it was by curating a visual display in a space which safeguarded confidentiality, as in Mahony (2010). I arranged the pictures chronologically to highlight the development of the work.

I spent time absorbing the display and making notes of my responses. I took photographs to make a visual record and database of the work. I recorded physical details of each picture, as well as title and date. My supervisors and fellow researchers visited the display and from different academic, psychodynamic and theoretical backgrounds made contrasting responses. This produced a broader base of ways to interrogate the meanings of the work, and highlighted how the meaning of visual material is affected by the way it is viewed and the context in which it is seen (Gilroy 2006; Rose 2001).

Findings and discussion

INITIAL OBSERVATIONS

Looking at the pictures without my clinical notes, it was as if I was at the exhibition of an artist (a different sort of viewer in a different context) and could bring more objectivity to the research. Instead of seeing the images under the influence of knowing what was going on in Alistair's life, I perceived other strands and an overall sense of Alistair's development.

Most of the work was 2D, with line drawing taking precedence over painting. The number of pictures produced at different periods in the therapy fluctuated to a marked degree, which invited investigation. I felt that the work could be divided into a series of distinct, stylistic phases which related to Alistair getting older and developing his understanding and artistic dexterity, but also to picture content and materials chosen. Unsurprisingly, through comparing my written data with the visual data, I found that these stages or stylistic groups often lined up with changes in Alistair's home situation or with changes at school. On the other hand, in the latter periods, there were times when my records state that Alistair was distressed outside the sessions but his artwork continued its flow without obvious distortion, as if the creative process had its own discrete momentum, and disturbance could be kept out to some degree.

By dividing the pictures into coherent groups, I was better able to study the function of the images and see how my patient adapted art-making for different purposes. It also helped me pick out pictures where regression to previous ways of working occurred and note the unusual, checking a picture against the relevant process notes.

Because of the brevity of this chapter, I will simplify my findings by discussing the artwork in terms of four phases, using one image to represent each 'group'.

FIRST PHASE

The first group comprises 27 paintings made over a period of six months. The pictures were notable in the display for being paintings rather than drawings, and for their spontaneity and experiment. They mark Alistair's arrival in school and belong to the period when Alistair was still living with his mother and was considered 'at risk' (see Figure 9.1).

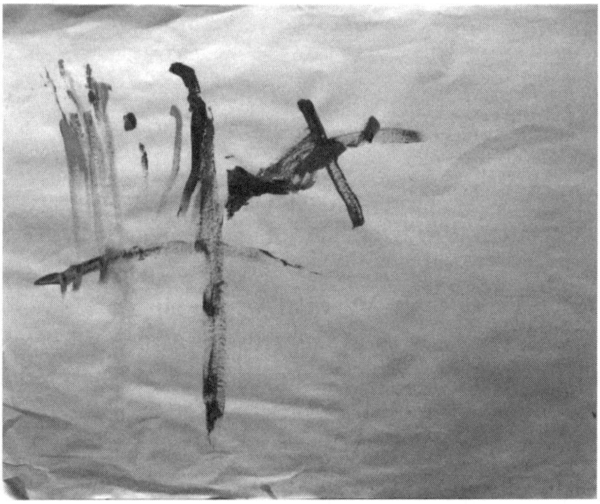

Figure 9.1: Crosses

The paintings appear to be non-figurative and there is interest in exploring what the brush can do, and discovery that marks can be placed in relation to each other. Far from being chance images, closer inspection reveals more intent on the part of the artist as time goes on, with, for example, marks placed carefully within circles (expressing a wish to be contained in psychodynamic terms). Figure 9.1, where crosses have been formed, was painted after a difficult playtime, and my notes indicate that Alistair's fast lines echo his movements in the room and contain emotion. Although he was testing boundaries in that session, he managed to make something coherent out of his feelings.

Overall, in these early paintings Alistair seems to be developing his sense of agency and capacity to order things; becoming familiar with the range of marks he can make and seeing his feelings made visible in them. This is a process often associated with pre-school children's first efforts to draw, which improves their understanding of how the world behaves and promotes the forming of ideas (Matthews 1999; Simon 1992). If Alistair had not had a reflective space to explore his world before, the calm of the art therapy room could provide what he had missed, and this appears to be a primary function of the image-making at this point, as well as helping him make a coherent product in the midst of his chaos. The art therapy literature supports the notion that the art process helps to repair developmental gaps (Meyerowitz-Katz 2003; Prokofiev 2010). There are proportionally fewer pictures in this group, but my notes show that he was also spending session time in sand and water play, which would give him other arenas in which to experiment with sensuous materials and explore his impact upon them.

SECOND PHASE

A new phase is introduced by a sudden end to exploratory painting in favour of felt-tip drawing, which offers more control, and a change to what looks like figurative work. This stylistic group covers four months, during which 66 pictures were made in twice-weekly art therapy. It coincides with Alistair's move into a hostel for looked-after children at five-and-a-quarter years old, and a time when he was reported to be distressed by any changes in class or the hostel. Letters, numerals and visual symbols, which are drawings round animals from the sand tray, are dispersed about the paper in many of the pictures in the four months following, but they are concrete objects, often haphazardly placed, rather than meaningful symbols; the letters are not formed into words and numerals intersperse with them. But Alistair is using society's languages and making them his own, and identifying more with his role as a schoolboy. My notes for one session tell me that Alistair was thrilled when I wrote his name and that I had to repeat this several times.

The pictures would be playful in their use of symbols if the drawn lines were not so faltering and vulnerable, which gives a desperate quality to their making.

In Figure 9.2 Alistair seems to be trying to get a grip on reality or pin it down somehow. He seems to be using the template as a prop, searching for something outside himself as support at this time when he is feeling so insecure and without his mother and attachment figure.

By the end of four months and this phase, the first images using a hesitant free hand are appearing: snowmen, a rainbow, and coloured circles

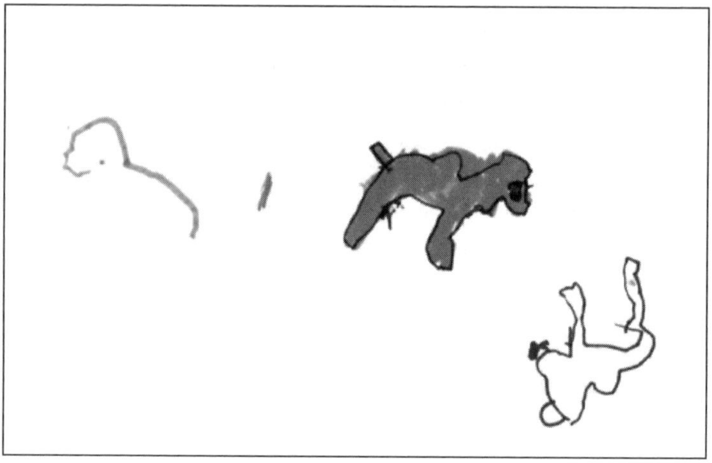

Figure 9.2: Capturing a 3D toy by outlining

one inside the other, painted with a fine brush. This represents more intentional thinking and the development of putting an idea on paper.

So the function of art-making as a stabilizing force at this unsettled stage is to offer Alistair a sense of having control and of building up defences. It appears that the art process has a function of actively supporting Alistair's transition into learning. More time was gradually being spent on art than play.

THIRD PHASE

The large group of pictures I am associating together here are more loosely connected and cover the long period from Alistair starting his second year at school, to the moment he left to go to a foster family nearly two years later. Although smaller subsections could be created, what links the pictures is that they have vivid imaginative subject matter and a confident and flowing style. There is a distinct divide between the end of the previous phase with its hesitancy, and the new beginning I call Phase 3. In this phase there is a return to spontaneity and freedom, but, with notable exceptions, not to using paint.

The number of pictures increases even more in Phase 3, and in the month Figure 9.3 was made there were no fewer than 72 pictures. Alistair's behaviour in the sessions showed how important art had become. He would enter the room asking for paper and make a start immediately, working with urgency until the end. Sometimes he might ask for 'something hard', as though he came with a feeling that needed a special kind of expression. He was single-minded, restarting an image more than once if it was not right, or starting with one idea that became another.

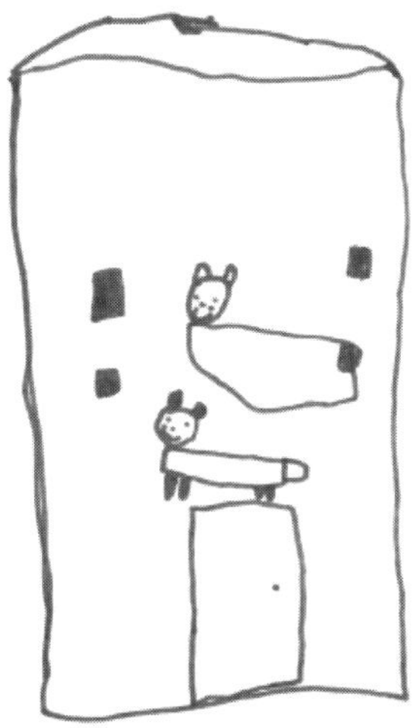

Figure 9.3 Two dogs in a house

Figure 9.3, 'Two dogs in a house', is the first of Phase 3 and part of a series with animals or dolphins, in and outside environments or swimming in waves composed of repeating letter 'Ms', which I relate to the ever-present 'Mum' in Alistair's mind. Alistair's mum was a central worry for him. Would she improve enough for the boys to return to her, or would they stay in the hostel forever? Could she manage without Alistair and his brother? Nine months later, one picture is an anguished letter to Mum, telling her of his love and wishes for her.

The most repeated theme in Phase 3 is Alistair's self-portrait: 77 portraits out of a total of 379 images, not including pictures of the letters of his name or creatures which represent him. He is often drawn side-by-side with his brother. Figure 9.4, made when Alistair was nearly six-and-a-half, is unusual in conveying what seems a sad, vulnerable image. The fact that he persisted with a scratchy pen when a stronger one could have been used suggests that this line conveyed his feelings at the time. Figure 9.5, by

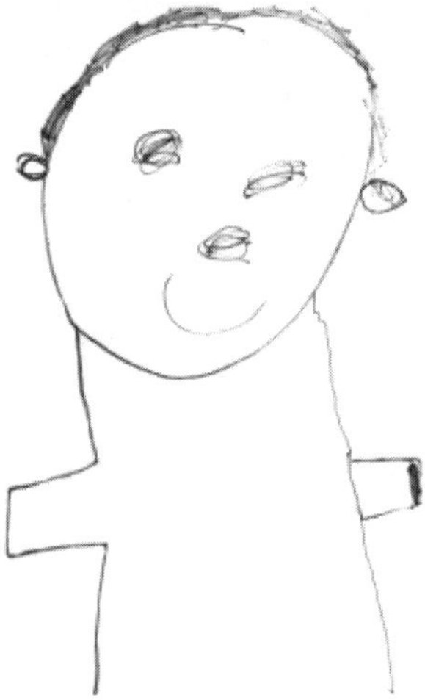

Figure 9.4: Self-portrait

contrast, drawn only two months later, presents two rather charming boys, where perfection seems looked for, with the ears of the first boy drawn round a circular template. The formula for drawing hair is a familiar one, where again the letter 'M' seems to lurk as if he cannot get 'Mum' out of his hair. When I looked at my notes for the session, I saw that it was drawn around the time that Alistair knew of the search for a long-term foster family; photographs of the brothers were taken to advertise them for this purpose. So perhaps his picture canvassed their appeal. Other portraits take the form of super-heroes (an aggrandized version of the self with strength to take on huge challenges?), and also full-size portraits which developed drawings he asked me to make round him as he lay on the floor.

Towards the end of the two-year period of Phase 3, there are four paintings made in a single session which seem to regress to the earliest phase of free painting. They were made on the day Alistair heard that foster parents had been found, and that he would be leaving the school and, as far as we knew then, ending art therapy. They express the conflicting feelings of relief and fear in outpourings of paint. My session notes reveal Alistair's shame about these pictures; he felt he was literally messing by exposing the feelings which he could not keep inside. Although he had been told he had the right to decide whether to move or not, at seven years old he had the insightfulness to tell me: 'I'll have to go; the point is, I haven't got a choice.'

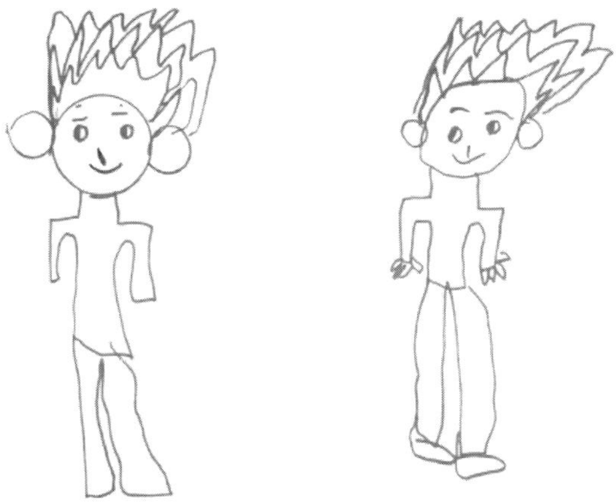

Figure 9.5: Two boys

So an important function of image-making as a stabilizing force in this phase includes putting unarticulated worries and preoccupations down on paper and exploring them creatively. Further factors include gaining a sense of coherence and relief, as well as having space for overwhelming feelings to be evacuated. Interpretations from me were still strongly resisted and only welcomed in Phase 4.

FOURTH PHASE

This group of pictures belongs to a discrete piece of art therapy work, created over the nine months at Alistair's new school after his move to a foster family. There is no space to do justice to the work here. I will simply point out that the subject matter changes, with many written references to his love for his new family, reflecting anxiety about whether he will be rejected. The artwork of this period is more sophisticated and includes portraits of his new family. Figure 9.6 shows him with his foster parents, as a replica of Dad in his efforts to identify with him and compete for the attention of his attractive new mum.

Artwork connected to the ending of art therapy shows new maturity in his thinking and inner world. Our dialogue was now more direct in putting words to his feelings, and interpretations were more acceptable.

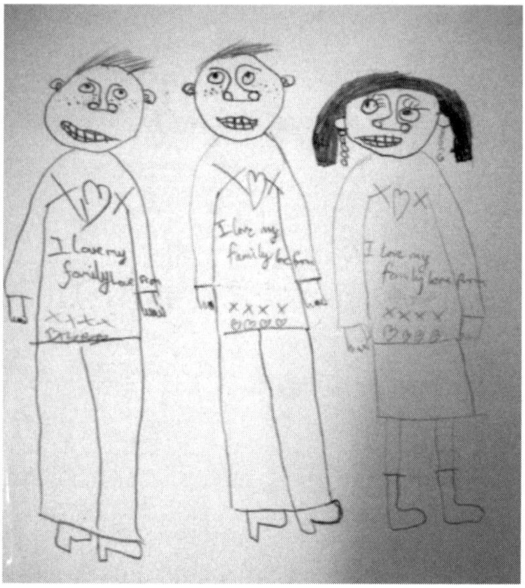

Figure 9.6: Alistair with foster parents

Discussion

Almost from the beginning of art therapy and certainly from Phase 2, there was no sign of the short attention span or poor fine motor control reported when Alistair started school. Art-making absorbed Alistair's interest, and he had the drive to pursue it in a focused way because he found meaning in the activity and it relieved his tension.

What is striking in Alistair's artwork is that despite his life challenges and emotionally deprived beginning, he was able to take risks and experiment rather than exercise such control that development was frozen. In Phase 2 it seemed that his ability to take risks was threatened, but he found a way to use art materials that was supportive and also expressive.

The periods of very industrious art-making are particularly intriguing. Searching the art therapy literature for examples of patients making more artwork when under particular stress produced some results in the area of trauma: Kalmanowitz and Lloyd (1997) offer an example when they describe urgent immersion in art-making in a group of refugee children who seem to go over their experience of trauma through 'making and re-making' as they come to terms with it (p.46). Case (1990), working in a short-term residential assessment centre where decisions were made about children's futures, describes a child who finds relief in the opportunity to immerse herself in messy paint and returns over and again to the art room to repeat the experience. It seems that when Alistair made his four messy paintings on hearing of his foster family, he was similarly using art-making in a fevered way to help him work through shocked feelings. To a less extreme degree it seems that he was using art to bring relief or regulate his feelings down to a manageable level throughout art therapy, and this supported his achievement of a modicum of normal development outside art therapy.

During Phase 3 Alistair showed enormous creativity in his artwork. In class he was concurrently becoming more able to cope with events such as his teacher being absent, without thinking it was because of him. Although he was in a group of low achievers in the class, he was within the range of normal development and did not need an Educational Statement of Special Needs, the government's recognition of the need for specialist help and extra funding.

The casework could not have been so successful without regular networking with experienced teachers who understood the meaning behind behaviour and offered understanding in the classroom on a daily basis.

CONCLUSION

This report has discussed the artwork of a single case study where a child with difficult beginnings and in the foster care system was able to progress developmentally despite losses and change.

I asked at the beginning how Alistair's image-making supported containment at a time of change and anxiety. In order to answer this I reviewed the images by investigating a retrospective visual display, which allowed me to assess the pictures in a new light as a whole body of work. The retrospective review proved a useful and appropriate methodology to clarify different functions of image-making.

My findings show that regular art therapy sessions, increased during a time of particular emotional pressure, enabled Alistair to use art for the discovery of meaning, self-exploration and emotional support. He was very young when art therapy began and, as Matthews (1999) suggests, the socio-cultural context of the first encounter with visual media is critical to the way in which the individual uses it in the future. Because art therapy was offered early on, Alistair is likely to have been best equipped to use it as a flexible tool. A child in a similarly precarious situation, beginning art therapy at a later age, might use art therapy differently.

It is worth considering whether findings from this case could be generalized to similar cases. As I suggest above, every aspect of the context influences how art therapy is used, and it is logical to suggest that the earlier the intervention, the better. This report shows that art therapy can support the regulation of unbearable feelings in children who have internalized few strategies to cope with crises and that because of this, offering art therapy during a period of transition can help a child to cope emotionally with the impermanence of their home situation. Key factors contributing to the value of art therapy in this context are that the focus is on the creative act, and that the art therapist is sensitive to the child's fear of direct interpretation.

REFERENCES

Aldridge, F. (1998) 'Chocolate or shit.' *Inscape 3*, 1, 2–9.

Bowlby, J. (1988) *A Secure Base: Clinical Applications of Attachment Theory.* London: Routledge.

Case, C. (1990) 'Reflections and Shadows: An Exploration of the World of the Rejected Girl.' In C. Case and T. Dalley (eds) *Working with Children in Art Therapy.* London and New York: Routledge.

Case, C. (2008) 'Playing Ball: Oscillations within the Potential Space.' In C. Case and T. Dalley (eds) *Art Therapy with Children: from Infancy to Adolescence.* London and New York: Routledge.

Gilroy, A. (2006) *Art Therapy. Research and Evidence-based Practice.* London: Thousand Oaks, CA and New Delhi: Sage Publications.

Hoxter, S. (1983) 'Some Feelings Aroused in Working with Severely Deprived Children.' In M. Boston, and R. Szur (eds) *Psychotherapy with Severely Deprived Children.* London: Routledge and Kegan Paul.

Kalmanowitz, D. and Lloyd, B. (1997) *The Portable Studio. Art Therapy and Political Conflict: Initiatives in Former Yugoslavia and South Africa.* London: Health Education Authority.

Mahony, J. (2010) 'Artefacts Related to an Art Psychotherapy Group: The Therapist's Art Practice as Research' In A. Gilroy (ed.) *Art Therapy Research in Practice.* Oxford: Peter Lang Publishing Group, forthcoming.

Matthews, J. (1999) *The Art of Childhood and Adolescence: The Construction of Meaning.* London and Philadelphia, PA: Falmer Press.

Meyerowitz-Katz (2003) 'Art materials and processes – a place of meeting. Art psychotherapy with a four-year-old boy.' *Inscape 8*, 2, 60–69.

O'Brien, F. (2008) 'Attachment Patterns through the Generations: Internal and External Homes.' In Case, C. and Dalley, T. (eds) *Art Therapy with Children: From Infancy to Adolescence.* London and New York: Routledge.

Prokofiev, F. (2010) '"I've Been Longing and Longing for More and More of This": Researching Art Therapy in the Treatment of Children with Developmental Deficits.' In A. Gilroy (ed.) (2010) *Art Therapy Research in Practice.* Oxford: Peter Lang Publishing Group, forthcoming.

Rose, G. (2001) *Visual Methodologies: An Introduction to the Interpretation of Visual Materials.* London: Sage.

Schaverien, J. (1991) *The Revealing Image: Analytical Art Psychotherapy in Theory and Practice.* London: Tavistock/Routledge.

Schaverien, J. (1995) 'The Retrospective Review of Pictures: Data for Research in Art Therapy.' In Payne, H. (ed.) *Handbook of Inquiry in the Arts Therapies: One River, Many Currents.* London and Philadelphia, PA: Jessica Kingsley Publishers.

Schore, A. (1994) *Affect Regulation and the Origin of the Self.* Hillsdale, NJ: Lawrence Erlbaum Associates.

Simon, R. (1992) *The Symbolism of Style, Art as Therapy.* London: Routledge.

Part II

Special Schools

Chapter 10

'I Am Here to Move and Dance with You'

Dance Movement Therapy with Children with Autism Spectrum Disorder and Pervasive Developmental Disorders

Hilda Wengrower

INTRODUCTION

Setting the scene

A number of children in special schools are diagnosed with some form of autism. Autism spectrum disorders (ASD) are 'characterized by varying degrees of impairment in communication skills, social interactions and restricted, repetitive and stereotyped patterns of behaviour' (ICD-10 2009; NIMH 2009). ASD comprises a range of specific diagnoses; autistic disorder is the severest of them. Other diagnoses included are Asperger syndrome, Rett Syndrome, and childhood disintegrative disorder. Autism is often used as a term to refer either specifically to the autistic disorder, or more generally to allude to a wide range of developmental deficits (ASD). Another term that is often used synonymously with ASD is 'pervasive developmental disorders' (PDD).

Some centres, like the Bloomberg School of Public Health at Johns Hopkins University, favour ASD over PDD because it highlights the shared, 'autism-like' quality of all of these specific diagnoses and reflects the broad range in the presentation of its characteristics. Others argue that individuals with PDD do not have enough, or severe enough, impairment in each of the characteristic ASD areas (social, communication, specialized interests) to warrant an autistic disorder diagnosis (Center for Autism and Developmental Disabilities Epidemiology 2009). In this chapter both terms will be used to refer to children with developmental difficulties with more or fewer autistic features.

Irrespective of the terminology used, dance movement therapists have been working with this population for years, thanks to their integration of nonverbal communication skills, their dance experience and acquaintance with psychology (Wengrower 2009). There is written and visual documentation of the contribution dance movement therapy (DMT) can make in producing changes in the three factors associated with autism mentioned above (i.e. difficulties with communication skills, social interactions and stereotyped patterns of behaviour; Adler 1968; Erfer 1995; Kalish 1968, 1977; Loman 1995; Tortora 2009).

Contemporary research in developmental psychology, as well as in neuropsychology, corroborates the importance of movement, dance and nonverbal communication in development as well as in therapy, thus adding other elements of knowledge that support our practice. There is also successful feedback between theories and propositions that arose from the psychodynamic psychotherapeutic setting, and from empirical research. Findings are giving validity to psychotherapy and add information that widens the clinical work, be it by mental health practitioners in general or dance movement therapists in particular (Alvarez 2004 (first published 1996); Greenspan and Wieder 1999, 2006; Subirana 2004; Tortora 2009; Viloca 2003, 2004).

There are several approaches to the psychotherapeutic treatment of ASD and PDD. Dance movement therapy (DMT) shares commonalities with the psychodynamic-developmental (Alvarez 2004/1996) and the developmental, individual difference, relationship-based model (DIR model) (Greenspan and Wieder 2006). All acknowledge that high cognitive abilities of language and thought, as well as emotional and social skills, develop in the frame of warm and meaningful relationships. Interpersonal communication and a sense of relatedness are seen simultaneously as pillars for child development and as the context where all other areas unfold towards integration, complexity and sophistication (Diamond 2001; Trevarthen and Aitken 2001). Dance movement therapists who have been working on this theoretical ground add to their multidisciplinary knowledge their fine scrutiny of the nonverbal, as framed in movement observation and evaluation systems such as Laban Movement Analysis, Kestenberg Movement Profile or Emotorics (Chaiklin and Wengrower 2009).

One of the basic techniques that has been used from the beginning, and is continually being refined, is what is called 'mirroring' or 'empathic reflection'. Developmental inquiry has recognized the role of imitation from the first moments of life, be it in typical or atypical growth. A review of research on this subject will be introduced, followed by a presentation of the parallel concepts and techniques in DMT and their applications in therapy with ASD and PDD.

LITERATURE REVIEW

Research on meanings and effects of imitation

Imitation used in various ways has been demonstrated to be an effective means of improving creative play, increasing interaction and attracting eye contact with the child with autism. Gaze behaviour, which is part of imitation, is a prelinguistic and social interaction milestone. Communication and early dyadic play include sharing gaze, building a dialogic closure, or dialogic space (Trevarthen *et al.* 1998). Malatesta and Izard (1984) argue that imitation aids the child to simultaneously see and feel emotion. We shall recognize later that the work of dance movement therapists is led by this idea, the use of mirroring or empathic reflection. They employ it without exerting pressure on the child, while enhancing their empathic attitude towards him or her.

Research has been carried out aiming to unveil the influence and meanings of imitation in typical and atypical development, as well as its effects in therapeutic interventions – although not as much as it deserves (O'Neill and Zeedyk 2006).

The varied difficulties children with ASD have in imitation are correlated with their impairment in social relations, being part of their intersubjective deficit and their limitations in reciprocal communication (Trevarthen *et al.* 1998). These researchers consider that the problems in imitation stem from their inability to form an internal image of the other as a partner in a mutual interaction 'with whom the child can explore how to share orientations to objects, exchange feelings about actions, objects and events and cooperate in performance of tasks' (Trevarthen *et al.* 1998, p.59). Nevertheless, Trevarthen *et al.* stated, these children do imitate and may be sensitive to the other's imitation of what they do. We shall see that further investigation, as well as DMT practice, has shown this as well.

For the sake of evaluating the effects of the adult imitating actions of typical children or of those with ASD, different situations have been created (i.e. various operative definitions have been established, as described below). Location for observation was mostly in a laboratory, less frequently at home.

Tiegerman and Primavera (1984) created a condition where the adult reproduced the child's play with a toy. They found that overall imitation generated eye contact from the children with ASD towards the adults. The best change in frequency and duration of gaze behaviour was obtained when the experimenter played with the same object as the child and duplicated his or her action with it.

Dawson and Galpert (1990) made a pre-test/post-test intervention with 15 pairs of children with autism and their mothers, interacting via imitative play mediated by toys. This included the possibility of imitating the child's movements and facial expressions. The treatment was carried out daily for 20 minutes a day over a two-week period. A majority of the children showed increased duration in holding gaze at the mother's face and improvement in creative play with toys, regardless of their personal developmental characteristics, IQ, ability to imitate or severity of autistic symptoms. After two weeks of treatment, children looked at mothers' faces and not at their play, leading to the conclusion that this interactive modality influences their interests in other people. Generalization to other situations remained to be established. Limitations of this research were: there was no follow-up after a significant time to establish the degree to which the effects were long-lasting; the number of participants was small; and participants were already enrolled in a comprehensive programme, which may have contributed to the positive results obtained.

Another study chose to avoid pre-structured interactions; the aim was to keep closer to the events in natural life. The researchers observed spontaneous, imitative exchanges in the play of children with developmental delay with adults (O'Neill and Zeedyk 2006). It was mostly the adults who initiated imitative bouts, and the children did not respond. But, following adults' imitations, they increased expressive-social communication through smile and vocalization, thus confirming their sensitivity to being imitated. One of the independent variables included was qualifying imitation into physical and vocalized actions. The former were successful in maintaining pre-existing behaviours that were already part of the dyad's repertoire, such as laughter, while the latter promoted increased eye contact.

All the papers mentioned report the use of imitation of the child for a short period of time, the longest being two weeks. In DMT, patients are seen for a longer time.

Jonsson, *et al.* (2001) consider that the means by which mothers naturally convey affect have clinical implications, as well as giving us information about development. As a result of research and that completed by others, it is possible to state that, through imitation, or parent's mirroring of affect (Jonsson *et al.* 2001), the child begins to be aware of his or her own emotions.

These investigators are not alone in extrapolating from normal development to children with autism (Trevarthen *et al.* 1998; Trevarthen and Daniel 2005).

> Given the retention of a degree of conscious awareness, every human being, even one handicapped by severe neuropsychological disorder, is sensitive at some level to the communicative expressions of other persons, and to the motives and emotions behind them. All humans are capable of detecting rhythmic impulses and qualities of other persons' behaviours that are contingent upon and related emotionally to their own expressions. These principles of fundamental intersubjectivity, which underlie but are not dependent on reason and language, are involved, though often not deliberately employed, in all therapeutic and educational procedures, just as they are continually present in family life and the daily activity of social groups. (Trevarthen and Aitken 2001, p.31)

Dance movement therapy with children with ASD: establishing a therapeutic relationship based on nonverbal communication

There is an exquisite video film that shows J. Adler's (1968) work with two girls with autism. One can see the gradual process in which the children begin to be aware of the therapist, and then allow her to share their personal space and change their isolated movement style into another with clear intersubjective quality. Their typical walking on tiptoes transforms into grounded strides.

Kalish (1968) was the first dance movement therapist to write a paper about her work with children with ASD, giving us information about how the embodied knowledge of a dance movement therapist, with her dance training and experience integrated with studies in psychology, guided her observations and practice. She stated that her initial goal was to try to establish a relationship with the child with ASD at the sensorimotor level, where he was primarily functioning. She did it by exploring with him body action, rhythm and vocalizations, hoping to create an emotional bond. In 1997, when being honoured by the Chace Foundation, Kalish remembered the psychoanalyst Dratman, who further articulated what she couldn't do before.

> [She] acts to help prevent the child from staying in the long sleep... [She] becomes involved with the child by using his movements as a bridge to elicit communication between them... The therapist takes the child where she finds him and...attempts to be his body double – with all his disturbance and his withdrawal – his autism...slowly she changes just one small part of the child's movements. She attempts to become part of the space and rhythm around him... (Kalish 1997, p.10)

Kalish was a student of Marian Chace, who, with her impressive intuition and dancer's knowledge, set many of the bases for DMT that were later developed by her apprentices and other colleagues. One of the fundamental principles of her work was highlighting the need to establish a therapeutic relationship through movement. In Chace's words: 'The movements used in establishing initial contact...may be qualitatively similar to those of the patient (not an exact mimicking since this is often construed by the patient as mocking)' (Chaiklin 1975, p.73). Or, as other disciples of Chace convey: '...she was able to incorporate the emotional content of the patient's behaviour into her own movement responses...reenacting the essential constellation of movement characterizing his expression' (Chaiklin and Schmais 1993 (first published 1979, pp.79–80).

Kalish calls 'mirroring' the act of adopting characteristics of the child's movement, and shares with the reader the delicacy of this communication: too much might cause the child to withdraw; too little or unclear might go unnoticed by the child. Also it is too difficult to do an exact mirroring. There is no need to replicate exactly the child's gestures; the therapist may sit at a distance tolerable for the child and give vocal, rhythmic expression to the rocking she witnesses. The therapist acknowledges the breathing and small, fleeting gestures. (A very interesting model of group work with children with autism and adults, based on breathing, was created by Blau and Siegel (1978).)

Kalish noted that in the group setting the children involved themselves more when the adults participating responded to (mirrored) their movements and were active in their communication. We can conclude that contact through mirroring and/or attunement was at the basis of the DMT therapy before the 1960s.

Imitation, mirroring and attunement, kinaesthetic empathy or empathic reflection

Some decades after Chace began to work in psychiatry and years after Adler and Kalish started their work with children with autism, Stern (1985) closely scrutinizes infant–mother rapport. He regards the sharing of affective states as an important feature of intersubjective relatedness that happens initially by means of the imitation the caregiver does of the infant's expression in his first months, and later develops into 'affect attunement'. Imitating is considered to be a fundamental feature of the first interchanges between adult and baby. Nevertheless, Stern considers that *strict* imitation (1985, p.139) won't really contribute to an exchange of feelings when babies are older (9–15 months old). This exchange can be achieved if the adult interprets the infant's feeling from his expression, and performs some behaviour that includes this understanding. The child has to be able to feel that there is some connection between the adult's reaction and himself.

The reader may recognise the similarity between this and the explanation of the work dance movement therapists do in order to communicate with their patients (as stated above). Stern calls this sharing 'attunement'. He describes it as a matching, an unplanned selection and recasting the adult does of some characteristics of the infant's expression, making some parallel pairing through a different channel of communication, spontaneously trying to get to the emotional core of the baby's state. For example, it may be that if the baby moves, the caregiver vocalizes the speed and energy of his movement, or gives a name and verbal description to what is happening (motor labelling). This was the type of work that Kalish engaged in, as mentioned earlier in this chapter.

Dance movement therapists know that it is almost impossible for an untrained person in a spontaneous interaction to perform *strict* imitation. Personal features of the imitator are always present, giving a special colour to this action. This is another reason why therapists do not make a straight connection between imitating or mimicking on the one hand,

and mirroring on the other. Loman (1998) distinguishes between *mirroring* (sharing or matching a similar body shape) and *attunement* (sharing or matching changes in muscle tension) as ways in which the dance movement therapist creates a relationship.

Sandel (1993) coins the term *empathic reflection* for the process by which the therapist incorporates parts of the client's expression and reacts to him or her in an empathic way. Chace talked about 'picking up' aspects from patients' expression in order to communicate with them. Those could be movement qualities or efforts, patterns, etc. (White 2009). The neologism of *mirroring* was later developed, and relates to part of the empathic process: it means trying to go into the other's experience, and not merely imitating him. This relies on a fine observation of the nonverbal, and of one's own body, movement awareness, and openness to one's sensations and feelings.

THE STUDY

The present paper offers a multiple case study, which consists of the presentation of parts of the narratives of three dance movement therapists as they wrote them in a case study, therapy diaries, and treatment reports of their work with children diagnosed with ASD or PDD.

The research question of the present study

As stated before, there are some constants over the years in the treatment of ASD using DMT. One of these is the concept of 'mirroring' (also referred to here as empathic reflection) and its application. On the other hand, developmental psychology research has also studied the role of 'imitation'. These two concepts, mirroring and imitation, appear fairly similar. Consequently, the question that guides this multiple case study is:

Although on first impression they might seem analogous, are there any differences between the definition and implementation of 'imitation' in developmental research studies, and of 'mirroring' in DMT? If yes, what are they?

Methodology

Multiple case study has been chosen as a design, since our interest is not in a particular case, but in examining how dance movement therapists work regarding a specific issue (Stake 1994; Yin 2003). In this case, the issue is to look at mirroring and empathic reflection and the connection there is between these therapeutic interventions and contemporary knowledge.

Much has been written about case studies and their status according to various methods of research. Due to space limitations I shall present the arguments that support my choice. Altogether case study has been appreciated for the possibility it allows us of entering into the intricacies of clinical work or of unique social situations. As Al Rubaie (2002) states, this method suits the research of psychotherapy, as it is a discipline dealing with the understanding and modification of the complexities of intra-psychic and interpersonal processes. It is also the professional's duty to attend to patients' particularities, as much as, or even more than, to their commonalities with some statistical norm.

The analysis employed was thematic, searching for sections of the therapists' notes that related to the use of mirroring or empathic reflection.

THE CHILDREN IN THIS MULTIPLE CASE STUDY

1. R. worked with Federico (all names have been changed), an eight-year-old child diagnosed with PDD, who lived in a warm and supportive family. He received medication to prevent epileptic seizures which he had at night. He had been treated in an orthopaedic service where he got a device to stretch his ankles and the posterior muscles of his legs. He had to increase the time of wearing it progressively. R and Federico met in the class for special education in a public mainstream school in the province of Barcelona. (Federico was in one of two special classes for children with ASD in the school.)

2. While doing her first year of internship, L. worked with Nicolas in a special education school in Northern Spain. He was eight years old, diagnosed with ASD. He was chosen because he showed some interest in L. during her observations at the classroom.

3. Antoni was sent to V. by a special education kindergarten when he was three years old. The professionals recommended to his parents a DMT process in order to work mainly on communication and interpersonal relations. He also received treatment at an Early Attention Centre. The parents were supportive and collaborative. V's work with this child was published (Villena Fresquet 2008).

Federico and Nicholas were seen at the schools they attended. Both children were selected for DMT together with their teachers. For Antoni, his school recommended that his parents take him to the private studio of the dance movement therapist, as there was no such kind of therapy as part of their services.

THERAPY ENVIRONMENTS

Some of the aspects the two therapists working in schools had to deal with were: to explain what DMT is; to establish a working and collaborative relationship with the school principal and the staff; and to create a suitable space for therapy. Neither of the two schools had experience of DMT before the therapists arrived. In both institutions they were received with curiosity, interest and openness.

Regarding allocation of an adequate space for the sessions: often, there is a lack of such room, as if the possibility of some movement activity that also requires intimacy had not been contemplated in the design of the school buildings (Wengrower 2001).

R. was offered the gymnasium, which was too big. She created a smaller space with benches. L. worked in what was called 'the psychomotor therapy room', which was actually used as a storeroom. She had to prepare it each day when she came to school. V. worked in her own studio, which was properly prepared.

All the therapists maintained communication with the children's teachers, exchanging relevant information about their process. In all three cases, their work was positively evaluated by the schools (Monsegur 2008).

Findings

We shall observe different uses and purposes of the technique of reflecting the child's movement. Many of the specificities of DMT have been left aside, due to the delimitated focus of this presentation.

REFLECTING THE CHILD'S MOVEMENT

1. Gaining attention and trust and leaving one's expectations aside

All the therapists used empathic reflection and mirroring in order to establish a therapeutic relationship with the child. The following narratives refer mainly to two themes:

> (a) *Mirroring and empathic reflection as a way to get the child's attention*
> Both L. and R. began with a period of participant observation in the classroom.
>
> L.: Mirroring was a fundamental tool for opening communication between us. My first purpose was to create a containing relationship. For this the child has to have an experience of being perceived, understood by me and then trusting and being interested in me.
>
> (b) *Learning the need for a paradoxical attitude*
> In order to 'succeed' and develop a relationship with the child, one has to be open and attentive to him, subduing one's own wishes to 'succeed'.

Although Nicolas established eye contact with L. when she mirrored him in the classroom, once they entered the space chosen to begin the DMT sessions, he didn't notice her, even when she mirrored him. More than this, he avoided her.

L. wrote:

> I felt anxious, wasn't sure about the suitability of reflecting these behaviours. I couldn't acknowledge Nicolas's anxiety due to the new situation: the room, [the intimacy of] our being together away from the others. He dealt with this by searching for material objects, ignoring me and wanting to leave the place.
>
> For me it was also my first DMT session, but I wasn't aware of my own wishes that all would go 'splendidly'. This was an important conclusion: the need to be sincere with myself and not pretend a tranquillity I wasn't feeling. Now I see I could have verbalized what I saw in myself and in him, to touch also the 'non-positive' feelings.
>
> From the second session, mirroring enabled us to make eye contact and exchange smiles. I initiate a ball game. He receives it, retains it and hits it, showing also that he wants to be in the room with the lights turned off. I accept. We bring some cushions from his classroom to the room where our encounters will take place. They seem to have the value of transitional objects [Winnicott 1971] and offer him a sense of safety, allowing him to take risks. The physical distance between us begins to shorten.

> Movement interactions involve whirling with hands clasped together, jumps and travelling along the room. This is followed by a characteristic expression of Nicolas: jumps and applauses. Then begins a second phase in the process when the boy looks for physical contact like being rocked and hugged, also hugging, hiding his face behind his shirt or behind my back. He goes over my face with the back of his hand. All this is mixed with some ambivalence, so it alternates with more distant movement playing.

R. described how Federico moved in circles about the room. She reflected the restraint and lightness characteristic of his movement, as well as describing verbally the motion and action of both. R. also clapped her hands, following Federico's rhythm: 'My goal was to establish a trusting relationship.' Nevertheless she felt that empathic reflection was frustrating her; he was totally disconnected, and after some sessions she began to feel anxious.

R. wrote:

> In supervision I became aware that the situation awoke in me my own fears of not being recognized...in spite of an apparently empathic attitude, I hoped he would come to me and do what I have thought in some way, for him.

R. remembered that these ritualistic actions had the power to soothe Federico until he could trust her (Viloca 2003). In supervision it was suggested to her to come to the sessions with a playful attitude...

> In the next session [the fifth], I decided to relax, do less and listen in order to attune with him. In the warm-up he already proposed movements without my asking for it...it developed into a playful warm-up and then into a movement dialogue.

V. was more experienced than her colleagues when she began to work with Antoni; she began to work with him after graduation. It was clear for her not only that when proposing something to him it should be developmentally and motivationally adequate to him, but also that *he* was the *protagonist:* 'I only had to accompany, to be present and contain' (Villena Fresquet 2008, p.4).

2. Mirroring helps get to know the child better because it allows for kinaesthetic empathy

> In DMT the nonverbal manifestations of the patient are fundamental for the evaluation of his needs and planning the treatment. For this, we observe him carefully, mirror his movements (moving like him, trying to breathe with him) in order to know him, empathize with him. (Villena Fresquet 2008, p.9)

R. wrote:

> While moving in circles like Federico, an image came to me of being on a track that gave me a sense of safety. Then I was reminded of the catastrophic anxiety of disappearing in a void that a child with PDD might experience.

3. Mirroring and empathic reflection create a shared playing space

During the seventh session, Nicolas rocked himself to and fro, and L. accompanied him in his movement.

> Suddenly he looked at me and began to laugh. Then he got up and jumped with another typical gesture of his, clapping his hands on his head and his back... Nicolas came to me, began to explore my forehead, kissed it (something he has been doing lately), laid himself on me; I rocked him all the time he allowed me. Then he jumped again, went to the hula hoops and took one, began to explore movements and play. I also took one and made the same movements; in addition I put it in front of him, made it spin and passed it over his head, so that Nicolas was inside the hula-hoop, and then made the reverse motion. This was repeated several times.

L. also mirrored Nicolas's play while he sat on a big ball: she squatted and jumped in front of him, sharing the rhythm and the height of the bounce. Nicolas laughed at this. When he stopped he extended his hands towards L., asking her in this way to whirl him, and this became a delightful moment of their sessions.

Discussion

Lack of the ability to imitate is considered a sign of autism (Landa 2007). Nevertheless, autistic children do imitate and are positively sensitive to being imitated, as has been shown in the studies described above, as well as in Field, *et al.* (2001). Even if they do not imitate, many of these children increase their interpersonal actions after being imitated. Most likely, the child finds interest in the adult's interest in him (Alvarez 2004/1996).

There are interventions that target the child's imitation, since it is considered a powerful tool for communication and a predictor for language acquisition (Landa 2007). However, in most of the studies reviewed there is an artificial flavour that involves repeating and reproducing.

As can be clearly understood from the writings of Chace (in Chaiklin 1975), Chaiklin and Schmaiss (1993/1979), Kalish (1968), Loman (1998) and Sandel (1993), dance movement therapists have made a clear distinction between mirroring and imitation; they sometimes call the latter 'mimicking'. The same definitions guided the three young therapists in this study, as has been witnessed from their writings. The purposes and results of using mirroring in DMT have much in common with those reported in this chapter so far, but there are also differences beyond what is imitated and how that imitation is used.

Research employed reproduction of the child's play with little toys; in one case it was repeating the rhythm played on a drum, and in many others the child was required to be seated at a table, while in DMT's sessions the child's needs are met respecting the place and posture adopted by him in the specific moment.

The reports analysed reveal that mirroring was used with different intentions and outcomes:

1. to establish a relationship that implies a sense of mutuality, attraction and interest towards the other
2. to know the child better and to empathize with him
3. to create a transitional space where play and bonding can evolve.

All of these intentions and outcomes were mediated by observation of the child's nonverbal expression, and the self-awareness of the therapist.

Probably the most interesting finding of this research is that mirroring or empathic reflection is not enough, no matter how well it is done. Both R. and L. came to sessions with a strong desire to succeed in their task, which, paradoxically, prevented them from being deeply attentive to the children's anxieties. It is not enough to try to pick up the patient's movement or to attempt to enter into his or her emotional state. The therapist has to be aware of her own anxieties and connected to her own feelings. This consideration takes us to Bion's concept of 'reverie' (1962) or to Winnicott's of 'holding' (1941): the attentive, receptive, introjective and experiencing quality that makes it possible to sustain uncertainty or the feeling of not knowing (Mitrani 2002).

R. also acknowledged her own fears of not being seen as a person. Once the therapists were aware of their own emotions, they could really be open to *seeing* the children and planting the seed of a relationship. From then on, their attitude changed. They could understand thoroughly the children's anxieties after bringing their own to supervision and receiving in return the verbal and empathic reflection of their supervisors and colleagues; they were contained by their supervision setting and helped to think.

CONCLUSIONS

Children with ASD or PDD are a strong challenge to people working with them. Dance movement therapists have a comprehensive knowledge of theories and techniques that allow them to reach those children. This is recurrently recognized by staff at the places where they work and it was the reason why the school took the initiative of sending Antoni to DMT with V.

The adult's imitation of the child's movements and actions has been found to have positive influences on normal children, as well as on those with ASD or PDD. As cited above, dance movement therapists have stressed the importance of incorporating the emotional content of the patient's behaviour. Tortora states:

> In mirroring, the therapist embodies the exact shape, form, and movement qualities of the child's actions, creating a mirror image of the mover. This qualitative matching includes depicting and connecting to the emotional expressivity of the child's movements. (Tortora 2009, p.166)

It seems that the therapist's anxieties, even when wishing very strongly to get the child's attention, may be a barrier to connecting with him in order to enter into his world. Empathy is not a magic or instant event arising from mirroring. It can be promoted by mirroring, but this is not totally assured. In the examples presented here, supervision and insight allowed the therapists really to express to the child: 'I am here to move and dance *with* you.'

ACKNOWLEDGEMENTS

I am very grateful to the therapists who generously allowed me to use their written material. They are: Edurne Calvo, Ester Bach and Olga Villena. Every therapy demands personal involvement. In order to respect their privacy I present their reports with an initial unconnected to their name, except for Olga Villena, whose work was published (2008). I want to acknowledge also Teresa Monsegur, with whom I shared the task of supervising these cases. I want to express my gratitude to Dr Beth Kalish for answering some questions regarding the history of her work and issues related to DMT and the treatment of ASD. I extend my thankfulness to Sharon Chaiklin for helping me to clarify historical aspects of the use of the term 'mirroring'; and finally, to Anne Wilson Wangh, who edited this English text.

REFERENCES

Adler, J. (writer/director) (1968) *Looking for Me.* (film) Berkeley, CA: Extension Media Center, University of California.

Al Rubaie, T. (2002) 'The rehabilitation of the case study method.' *European Journal of Psychotherapy, Counselling and Health 5,* 1, 31–47.

Alvarez, A. (2004) 'A propósito del elemento de déficit en niños con autismo.' In J. Brun and R. Villanueva (eds) *Niños con Autismo.* Valencia: Promolibro (First published in 1996 as 'Addressing the element of deficit in autism: psychotherapy which is both psychoanalytically and developmentally informed.' *Clinical Child Psychology and Psychiatry 1,* 4, 525–537.)

Bion, W.R. (1962) 'A theory of thinking'. *International Journal of Psycho-Analysis 43,* 306–310.

Blau, B. and Siegel, E. (1978) 'Breathing together: a preliminary investigation of an involuntary reflex as adaptation.' *American Journal of Dance Therapy 2,* 1.

Bloom, K. (2006) *The Embodied Self.* London: Karnac.

Center for Autism and Developmental Disabilities Epidemiology (2009) 'Autism factsheet. John's Hopkins University, Bloomberg School of Public Health. Available at www.jhsph.edu/CADDE/Facts/autism.html, accessed on 28 April 2009.

Chaiklin, H. (ed.) (1975) *Marian Chace: Her Papers.* Columbia, MD: *ADTA.*

Chaiklin, S. and Schmais, C. (1993) 'The Chace Approach to Dance Therapy.' In S. Sandel, S. Chaiklin and A. Lohn (eds) *Foundations of Dance/Movement Therapy.* Columbia, MD: 'The Marian Chace Memorial Fund.' (First published 1979 in P. Lewis Bernstein (ed.) *Eight Theoretical Approaches in Dance-Movement Therapy.* Dubuque, IA: Kendall/Hunt.

Chaiklin, S. and Wengrower, H. (eds) (2009) *The Art and Science of Dance Movement Therapy. Life is Dance.* New York/London: Routledge.

Dawson, G. and Galpert, L. (1990) 'Mothers' use of imitative play for facilitating social responsiveness and toy play in young autistic children.' *Development and Psychopathology,* 2, 151–162.

Diamond, N. (2001) 'Towards an interpersonal understanding of bodily experience.' *Psychodynamic Counselling 7,* 1, 41–62.

Erfer, T. (1995) 'Treating Children with Autism in a Public School System.' In F. Levy (ed.) *Dance and Other Expressive Therapies. When Words Are Not Enough.* London: Routledge.

Field, T., Field, T., Sanders, C. and Nadel, J. (2001) 'Children with autism display more social behaviors after repeated imitation sessions.' *Autism 5*, 3, 317–323.

Greenspan, S. and Wieder, S. (1999) 'A functional developmental approach to autism spectrum disorders.' *The Journal of the Association for Persons with Severe Handicaps 24*, 3, 147–161.

Greenspan, S. and Wieder, S. (2006) *Engaging Autism.* Cambridge, MA: Da-Capo.

ICD–10 (2009) 'Pervasive Developmental Disorders and Autism.' Available at www.who.int/classifications/apps/icd/icd10online/, accessed on 28 January 2009. Geneva: World Health Organization.

Jonsson, C., Clinton, D., Fahman, M., Mazzaglia, G., Novak, S. and Sörhus, K. (2001) 'How do mothers signal shared feeling states to their infants? An investigation of affect attunement and imitation during the first year of life.' *Scandinavian Journal of Psychology 42*, 4, 377–381.

Kalish, B.I. (1968) 'Body movement therapy for autistic children: a description and discussion of basic concepts.' *Journal of the American Dance Therapy Association 1*, 1, 7–9.

Kalish, B. (1977) 'Body movement therapy for autistic children.' *Focus on Dance,* 48–59.

Kalish, B. (1997) 'Through dance/movement therapy to psychoanalysis.' Marian Chace Foundation Lecture. *American Journal of Dance Therapy 19*, 1, 5–14.

Landa, R. (2007) 'Early communication development and intervention for children with autism.' *Mental Retardation and Developmental Disabilities Research 13,* 1, 16–25.

Loman, S. (1995) 'The Case of Warren: A KMP Approach to Autism.' In F. Levy (ed.) *Dance and Other Expressive Art Therapies.* New York: Routledge.

Loman, S. (1998): 'Employing a developmental model of movement patterns in Dance/Movement Therapy with young children and their families.' *American Journal of Dance Therapy 20*, 2, 101–115.

Malatesta, C. and Izard, C.E. (1984) 'The Ontogenesis of Human Social Signs. From Biological Imperative to Symbol Utilization.' In N.A. Fox and R.J. Davidson (eds) *The Psychobiology of Affective Development.* Hillsdale, NJ: Erlbaum.

Monsegur, T. (2008) 'Testimonios de los profesionales en los centros donde se ha introducido la DMT.' In H. Wengrower and S. Chaiklin (eds) *La Vida es Danza. El Arte y la Ciencia de la Danza Movimiento Terapia.* Barcelona: Gedisa.

Mitrani, J.L. (2002) 'Replies to questionnaire.' *Journal of Analytical Psychology 47*, 47–56.

NIMH (2009) 'Autism Spectrum Disorders (Pervasive Developmental Disorders).' Available at www.nimh.nih.gov/health/topics/autism-spectrum-disorders-pervasive-development-disorders/index.shtml

O'Neill, M. and Zeedyk, M. (2006) 'Spontaneous imitation in the social interactions of young people with developmental delay and their adult carers.' *Infant and Child Development 15*, 3, 283–295.

Sandel, S. (1993) 'The Process of Empathic Reflection in Dance Therapy.' In S. Sandel, S. Chaiklin and A. Lohn (eds) *Foundations of Dance/Movement Therapy: The Life and Work of Marian Chace.* Columbia, MD: Marian Chace Foundation.

Stake, R. (1994) 'Case Studies.' In N. Denzin and Y. Lincoln (eds) *Handbook of Qualitative Research.* Thousand Oaks, CA: Sage.

Stern, D., (1985) *The Interpersonal World of the Infant.* New York, NY: Basic Books.

Subirana, V. (2004) 'El Juego en los Niños con Trastorno Autista.' In J. Brun and J. Villanueva (eds) *Niños con Autismo. Experiencia y experiencias.* Valencia: Promolibro.

Tiegerman, E. and Primavera, L. (1984) 'Imitating the autistic child: facilitating communicative gaze behaviour.' *Journal of Autism and Developmental Disorders 14*, 27–38.

Tortora, S. (2009) 'Dance Movement Psychotherapy in Early Childhood Treatment.' In S. Chaiklin and H. Wengrower (eds) *The Art and Science of Dance Movement Therapy: Life is Dance.* New York: Routledge. (In Spanish: 'La Danza Movimiento Terapia en el tratamiento de niños pequeños. Diferentes puntos de vista.' In H. Wengrower and S. Chaiklin (eds): *La Vida es Danza. El Arte y la Ciencia de la Danza Movimiento Terapia.* Barcelona: Gedisa.)

Trevarthen, C. (1979) 'Communication and Co-operation in Early Infancy: a Description of Primary Intersubjectivity.' In M. Bullowa (ed.) *Before Speech.* Cambridge: Cambridge University Press.

Trevarthen, C., Aitken, K., Papoudi, D. and Robarts, J. (1998) *Children with Autism: Diagnosis and Interventions to Meet Their Needs.* London, Jessica Kingsley Publishers.

Trevarthen, C. and Aitken, K.J. (2001) 'Infant intersubjectivity: research, theory, and clinical applications.' *Journal of Child Psychology and Psychiatry 42,* 1, 3–48.

Trevarthen, C. and Daniel, S. (2005) 'Disorganized rhythm and synchrony: Early signs of autism and Rett syndrome.' *Brain and Development 27,* 1, 25–34.

Villena Fresquet, O. (2008) 'Una experiencia de DMT con un niño con trastorno multisistémico del desarrollo. Terapia a través del movimiento y la danza.' Special dossier in *Babel, Revista de Psicología de la Universidad Bolivariana de Chile.* Available at http://www.revistababel.cl/6/indice.htm, accessed on 28 January 2009.

Viloca, L. (2003) *El Niño autista.* Barcelona: CEAC.

Viloca, L. (2004) 'Incidencia de la Ansiedad Catastrófica el Desarrollo Emocional y Cognitivo de Niños Autistas.' In J. Brun and J. Villanueva (eds) *Niños con Autismo. Experiencia y experiencias.* Valencia: Promolibro.

Wengrower, H. (2001) 'Arts therapies in educational settings: an intercultural encounter.' *The Arts in Psychotherapy 28,* 2, 109–115.

Wengrower, H. (2009) 'The Creative Artistic Process in Dance Movement Therapy.' In S. Chaiklin and H. Wengrower (eds) *The Art and Science of Dance Movement Therapy. Life is Dance.* New York: Routledge. (In Spanish: 'El proceso creativo y la actividad artística por medio de la danza y el movimiento.' In H. Wengrower and S. Chaiklin (eds) (2008) *La Vida es Danza. El Arte y la Ciencia de la Danza Movimiento Terapia.* Barcelona: Gedisa.)

White, E. (2009) 'Laban's Movement Theories. A Dance/Movement Therapist's Perspective.' In S. Chaiklin and H. Wengrower (eds) *The Art and Science of Dance Movement Therapy. Life is Dance.* New York: Routledge.

Winnicott, D.W. (1941) 'The Observation of Infants in a Set Situation.' In *Collected Papers: Through Paediatrics to Psychoanalysis.* New York: Basic Books.

Winnicott, D.W. (1971) *Playing and Reality.* London: Penguin.

Yin, R.K. (2003) *Case Study Research. Design and Methods.* Thousand Oaks: Sage.

Chapter 11

Dramatherapy, Autism and Relationship Building: A Case Study

Lynn Tytherleigh and Vicky Karkou

INTRODUCTION

Setting the scene

The *Shorter Oxford Dictionary* (1993) defines 'relationship' as 'an emotional association between two people'. Clarkson (1994) describes relationship as 'the interconnectedness between two people' or 'the betweenness of people' (p.29). She adds that 'relationship is the first condition of being human' (p.29). The underlying assumption of this position is that humans are fundamentally social beings, and that as such they strive for connection and communication with another and/or others.

The idea of humans, and infants in particular, being inherently social departs from perceptions of development within early psychotherapeutic thinking that highlight either instinct (as in Freudian thinking) or pleasure (see Kleinian work) as key factors guiding growth. Within a perspective that stresses the social aspects of human nature, infants are seen as driven by the need to communicate with others and be with them. Trevarthen *et al.* (1998), for example, describe infants' first few months of life as the time when they form relationships with caregivers, through 'primary intersubjectivity' and the rhythmic turn-taking of expressive acts. From around nine months joint 'secondary intersubjectivity' develops, this term stands for shared attention, directed by both carer and child together towards an external object (Trevarthen *et al.* 1998).

However when it comes to children with autism, things can be very different. Hobson (2007), for example, believes that children with autism are impaired in primary and secondary intersubjectivity, having difficulties with making connections with others, identifying with others, or even allowing others to have any effect on them.

Despite apparent difficulties in relating, evidence suggests that many people with autism do respond to others, care what they feel, and form attachment relationships and friendships with others (Cesaroni and Garber 1991; Hobson 2007). Noble (2001) adds that many children with autism are motivated to make and keep friends if they have not already been overwhelmed with a sense of social failure and rejection. Blotzer (1995), drawing on her psychotherapeutic work with people with autism, asserts that her clients crave connection with other people and want to be deeply understood. However, this has to be in a form that is tolerable to them. Writings from people with autism support this idea. For example, Williams (1996), herself a person with autism, describes what she terms sensory experience-based relationships, explaining as an example how she relates to her husband partly as a collection of sensory experiences.

Because of the differences and consequent difficulties in forming relationships, supporting ways in which people, and children in particular, with autism relate with others can become particularly important. According to Greenspan and Wieder (1997), the interactions that a child with autism has in different types of relationships form a main vehicle for enabling development and growth. This chapter will focus on different types of interactions that took place within six dramatherapy sessions with children with autism. We will make links between these interactions and relationship building. Furthermore, based on this brief therapeutic intervention, we will make some tentative suggestions about the potential contribution of dramatherapy towards relationship building with this client group.

LITERATURE REVIEW

What can we learn from existing interventions?

Interventions that focus on interaction, communication and relationships when working with children with autism are wide-ranging, highlighting slightly different aspects of work. For example, within a psychodynamic frame, the Tavistock autism team (Alvarez and Reid 1999; Alvarez, Reid and Hodges 1999) stress the role of the relationship between client and therapist, suggesting that this enables the child to form better relationships with others. They note that it is the emotionality in the contact which promotes change in social relatedness, stating that the therapist may actively need to reclaim the child back into the world of human relatedness, and demonstrate that the world outside their own autism is interesting (Alvarez and Reid 1999).

Others argue for the value of play as part of 'normal' development (Stern 1985; Vygotsky 1978) that can also be introduced to working with autism (Janert 2000; Wieder and Greenspan 2003). Janert (2000), for example, describes how adult–child play and games resembling those that parents naturally engage in with typically developing infants and young children can reach the communicative, non-autistic potential of young children with autism. She stresses the importance of meeting the child where they are at, and of the need for shared pleasure in the play.

Stressing the importance of play, Wieder and Greenspan (2003) write:

> In children with autistic spectrum disorders, interactive play uniquely addresses the core deficits of relating and communicating as no other approach can. (2003, p.426)

Play therapists Bromfield (1992), Josefi and Ryan (2004), and Mittledorf, Hendricks and Landreth (2001) report success in building therapeutic relationships with children with autism using individual, child-led play therapy.

Closely connected with play therapy is the contribution made by arts therapists. There are interesting accounts of building therapeutic relationships with children with autism in music (Alvin 1978; Brown 2002; Robarts 1996; Turry and Marcus 2003; Woodward 2004), art therapy (Evans and Dubowski 2001), and dance movement therapy (Kalish 1968; Loman 1995; Parteli 1995). Within the arts therapies literature, some authors stress the value of the arts as ways in which children develop their sense of self, awareness of others and social skills (Lord 2000; Noble 2001). In order to achieve these, arts activities need to maintain each child's interest and be developmentally appropriate. Noble (2001) also refers to the importance of vigilance to the group's varying needs for structure, and for the therapist's patience and flexibility in the face of individuals' high anxiety and group chaos. Furthermore Noble (2001) suggests that individual activities may provide a needed rest from the stress of relating to others. These are useful guidelines for practice that have informed the dramatherapy intervention described in this chapter.

Also relevant to this chapter and the dramatherapy intervention adopted with this client group is the developmental, individual difference, relationship-based model (DIR model), proposed by Wieder and Greenspan (2003). The model is based on an understanding of the developmental capacities that emerge during childhood, individual differences or deficits which need support, and the relationships and interactions necessary to enhance, nurture and practise the emotional, social and cognitive capacities of the child. An essential part of this holistic support is daily 'floor time' or interactive play sessions with an adult. Within the sessions children are guided through developmental levels of play, from self-regulation and shared attention at Stage 1 towards building bridges with symbols at Stage 6. In floor time, at each level, through spontaneous play, the adult responds to the child's lead, encouraging a 'continuous flow of interactions utilizing affect cues that entice, challenge, soothe and encourage the child further' (Wieder and Greenspan 2003, p.427).

Dramatherapy, relationships and learning difficulties

A wide range of activities can fall under 'dramatherapy' including movement and dance. Sherborne's developmental movement (2001) can be particularly useful, as it offers a developmental frame that can support communication and relationships. Through 'caring', 'shared' and 'against' relational movement with a caregiver, Sherborne (2001) argues that the child can experience security, learn to trust and communicate, and gain confidence. Wethered (1993) refers to the developmental movement work of Sherborne, noting that people can experience the inner flow of relationship through interchange of mutual support and reliance on other people.

Jennings (1990, 1993, 1999, 2006) also offers a developmental perspective on working with clients and embraces the whole range of dramatherapy artistic media. Jennings' model is known as the 'embodiment, projection and role' (EPR) model. Embodiment play is most prominent from 0–14 months, including sensory experiences such as holding, whole-body and body-part activities, touch, massage, singing games and 'peep-bo'. Jennings (1990, 1993), for example, proposes that Sherborne's developmental movement is a valuable example of embodiment activity. Jennings' *projective* stage (from 15 months to 3–4 years) is 'beyond the body' when the infant plays with sand, water toys, puzzles, art materials, puppets and the doll's house. In the more complex *role* stage (4–7 years) the child is able to dramatize a character and scene and take on the role of another.

Jennings (1983) notes the importance of children being given the chance to navigate through all three play stages in therapy if they have not had these primary experiences in their first years of life. This is particularly relevant for people with autism, who may not have passed through the typical developmental stages (Jordan 2003).

The EPR paradigm is implicit in Chesner's model for dramatherapy with people with learning difficulties. Chesner (1995) uses an integrated model with learning disabilities that incorporates dance and movement, art, music-making, contact exercises, games, storymaking, role-play and performance. This multimodal aspect of dramatherapy can provide a range of opportunities to make contact with individuals with autism. A familiar structure of warm-up, exploration and closure is suggested to provide the ritual that develops trust and a sense of security (Chesner 1995; Jennings 1990). This is particularly valuable for many people with autism who find unpredictable and open-ended situations stressful.

Dramatherapy with people with autistic spectrum disorder

In 2004 when this study took place, very little was written on dramatherapy with people with autism (e.g. Carrette 1992; Jones 1984, 1996; Lindkvist 1997). More recently Miller (2005) and Crimmens (2006) have offered valuable accounts of group dramatherapy, while Jones (2007) offers an insightful description of individual work.

Some of the key themes dealt with in the reviewed literature are summarized here. Carrette (1992), for example, attempts to show that the flexibility of dramatherapy can help to address identified areas of difficulty in a person with autism. Carrette (1992) notes that, while what is achievable will be different for each child with autism, most will work at the basic movement end of the spectrum.

Similar emphasis seems to be placed on movement work by Lindkvist (1997) who gives examples of how, in a dramatherapy group, one-to-one relationships were developed as members of the therapeutic team communicated in playful ways with clients in the clients' own movement activity. However, the success cited by Greenspan and Wieder (1997) and Wieder and Greenspan (2003), using the DIR model, suggests that many children with autism are also capable, with effective intervention, of working towards the role end of the spectrum. Crimmens (2006), for example, offers opportunities for groups of students with autism to take on roles in enacting stories, supported by the use of props and storyboards.

Another interesting aspect of work coming from the reviewed literature is the degree to which one-to-one or group relationships can be developed with this client group. Miller (2005) describes some success in the development of group relationships amongst children with pervasive developmental disorders, including autism. She uses an interesting combination of group dramatherapy and friendship skills training, which could be valuable for children with more advanced social skills and experience in groups other than those in the present study. Still, Miller's (2005) example brings to the foreground the need to explore further the potential capacity of children with autism to relate at a group level.

THE STUDY

Aim and research questions

This chapter draws upon six sessions of dramatherapy held weekly with two 11-year-old children with autistic spectrum disorder. Although it was a particularly small number of participants, the sessions were treated as group sessions that consisted of the two children, the first author (Lynn) in her role as a dramatherapist, and the children's class assistant. The group had a clear aim: to offer opportunities for building relationships. For the purposes of the study, an overall exploratory ethos was adopted that aimed to answer the following two questions:

- *Were relationships built in this group?*
- *If so, how was their development supported?*

Methodology

According to Grainger (1999), there is no external, objective rule we can use to measure the quality of human relationship. As relationships are difficult to quantify, this study was naturally conceptualized within the qualitative paradigm that valued personal perspectives, and was primarily process-oriented. It was expected that an in-depth study of the therapist's and the clients' experiences of the particular dramatherapy group would offer an understanding of the therapeutic work, improve therapeutic interventions and skills, and potentially suggest ways in which dramatherapy could support relationship building with this client group. These reasons led to choosing a case study as the preferred research design.

Case studies have been criticized for bias and lack of ability to generalize from the findings (Yin 2003). In response to this, Yin (2003) argues that there is a need for all researchers to avoid biases; this includes both the qualitative and the quantitative researcher. Ways in which this can be achieved within a case study are through reporting evidence fairly, and making sure that all procedures are transparent and clear. Regarding generalizability, Yin (2003) argues that because of the small sample usually included in case studies, one can generalize to *theoretical propositions* and not to populations. In other words, findings from a case study can contribute towards developing, expanding and/or refining theory. Identifying what is specific and unique on the one hand, and on the other what might be potentially transferable to other situations, is a key feature of case studies, and consequently relevant to this study.

As a case study looks at collecting information from a number of different sources in a number of different ways, in this study the following methods were used:

- participant observation
- observation of video recordings of sessions
- observation of clients outside sessions
- reflection with the co-worker and clients
- discussion with the class teacher and clients' parents.

The group process was described and analysed, focusing on *significant events*. This method is adapted from the work of Elliot and Shapiro (1992), according to whom 'significant events represent important general therapeutic factors but in more concentrated form' (p.164). In this study significant events were defined as verbal and nonverbal interactions that might suggest development of relationship between two or more people. Significant events were selected by the dramatherapist (Lynn, the first author), based on her experience with the clients in therapy, on discussion with the co-worker, and on observation of video recordings of the sessions. An experienced music therapist assisted the analysis of the events by observing and reflecting on video recordings. This reinforced the concept of *intersubjectivity*, i.e. a shared, subjective view of the accuracy and value of the findings. Intersubjectivity became important as an alternative to *objectivity* within a research frame (Ansdell and Pavlicevic 2001), but was also seen as particularly relevant to human development (Stern 1985; Trevarthen *et al.* 1998), therapy (Grainger 1999), and so as central to this study that looked at the formulation of relationships within dramatherapy for children with autism.

The school setting

In the school for children with learning difficulties in which this study took place, students with a high degree of autism were taught together, using the Division TEACCH (Treatment and Education of Autistic-related Communication-handicapped CHildren) approach (Schopler and Olley 1982). As a result of following this approach, for most of the day the pupils worked on highly structured individual tasks with little time spent interacting with other pupils.

Newly appointed to introduce dramatherapy to the school, the first author, Lynn, was requested to facilitate six-week blocks of dramatherapy with each class in Key Stage 3. It was felt that, although the intervention was particularly short, it would give clients the opportunity to experience working together in dramatherapy, and help to identify those clients who might benefit most from a longer period of dramatherapy.

After discussion with teachers and classroom observations, one class of seven children was selected for dramatherapy. The class was divided into two groups (of two and five), as a way of addressing the fact that two of the children seemed much more withdrawn and appeared to be intimidated by their boisterous classmates. Both groups received dramatherapy. Here, we will focus on the work carried out with the two children only.

The intervention

The group met weekly in a room free from distracting sensory stimuli. The first session lasted 30 minutes, and the remaining five sessions were extended to 40 minutes, which was the maximum time available within the school timetable.

An overall developmental approach was followed that was informed by the embodiment, projection, role (EPR) model (Jennings 1990, 1993, 1999), and the multi-modal work of Chesner (1995) in dramatherapy with people with learning difficulties. Influences from the developmental movement work of Sherborne (2001) were also present.

Each session followed a similar structure to provide security and limit anxiety, as argued in the relevant literature (Chesner 1995; Crimmens 2006; Jennings 1990; Noble 2001). In most sessions small variations and new methods were introduced within the structure. Sessions began with a 'story of the circle' dance (Brigg 1996) that involved holding hands in a circle. The 'story of the circle' aimed to welcome each individual, encourage awareness of one another and establish a feeling of togetherness. This was followed by group games with a ball, aiming to develop social awareness: turn-taking, joint attention and communication. Next, each adult partnered a client, offering activities to develop trust and relationships. Developmental movement activities with a partner were introduced at the beginning, and were at times replaced with improvized games. Pretend play with balls and beanbags was introduced in Session 4 and used subsequently. Sessions ended with a group activity such as 'story of the circle' or a ball game, selected by the clients, and with reflection. During reflection time clients were asked which activities they liked the most and which they disliked. This was aided by a set of cards with pictures of the activities and a blank card in case a client wished to choose nothing.

Findings and discussion

THE CHILDREN

The children participating in this study (we shall call them Jenny and Tim) did not relate to their peers, and avoided group activities. Jenny would protest loudly and require much time and persuasion before she would join a group. Tim was often in a world of his own, reciting events from *Thunderbirds* or imitating radio disc jockeys. He rarely related to his peers, or to staff, unless to ask for something. He often refused to do what others asked him to do, such as his work tasks. He did not join in group activities. In P.E. lessons he would stand by the wall or in a corner, saying 'No'.

SIGNIFICANT EVENTS

Following Elliot and Shapiro's (1992) conceptualization of *significant events*, particular attention was paid to (1) the context of the event, (2) the important features of the event, and (3) its impact.

The significant events selected and presented here refer first to each client separately and second to the group as a whole. Relevant reflections and discussion with regard to the literature are included.

One-to-one relationship with Jenny

Building relationships through embodiment play – 'relaxing with Diane'

Jenny (aged 11) joined in all of the activities only tentatively at first. However, as early as the first session Jenny responded positively to the offer of lying on the lap of the class assistant (whom we will call Diane). In the therapist's notes of the first session we find the following comments describing this first significant event:

> In partner work Jenny enjoyed relaxing on Diane's lap, being cradled, and asked to repeat this. Jenny found this so pleasurable [that] she initially said 'No' to the next activity, which was 'Row your boat'. Finally she sat facing Diane, rowed back and forward singing, and then said 'Night night', indicating she wanted to lie on Diane's lap again. (Therapist's clinical notes, Session 1)

Following this session Jenny often talked excitedly about 'drama' and 'relaxing with Diane', and this became her favourite part of every session.

It appeared that the relationship between Jenny and Diane began through the use of early 'developmental movement', and in particular the type of relationship that Sherborne (2001) referred to as a 'caring' type. We have already discussed Sherborne's developmental movement as being closely linked with Jennings' (1990, 1993, 1999, 2006) 'embodiment play', the first developmental stage within her EPR model. Diane responded to Jenny's lead while gently encouraging Jenny to try a number of different activities. The initial 'relaxing with Diane', cradling and rocking, gradually developed into games where each partner would pretend to sleep, and be awakened by gentle tickling.

Cesaroni and Garber (1991) stress the importance of recognizing the strong need for human contact that people with autism experience, despite their unusual behaviours. It is possible that, through being cradled, Jenny was able to feel contained and supported by her partner. Being cradled can also have direct associations with sensory experiences that are extensively discussed within the autism literature. Williams (1996), for example, describes sensory experience-based relationships, noting that people often try to train people with autism out of relating to people as sensory experiences – the result sometimes being that they end up feeling nothing at all. She suggests that it would be better to support people with autism to restrict indulgence in sensory experience to certain environments or times. Dramatherapy provided a good opportunity for Jenny to develop a sensory experience-based relationship with Diane.

Building relationships through projection – 'the dog game with Lynn'

In Session 5 Tim was absent, so Jenny and Lynn worked alone together. Jenny declined Lynn's suggestions to engage in activities without an object between them. Finally she chose playing with a ball. In Jennings' (1990, 1993, 1999, 2006) EPR model, the use of objects can be seen as closely connected with projection, the second stage of Jennings' understanding of development. Furthermore, Alvin (1978), in music therapy, describes how, when working with children with autism, the use of objects is particularly relevant to making intimacy bearable. Consequently the object encapsulates aspects of the relationship. In this case, the ball may have played this role, as presented in the following significant event.

> After some play with the ball, Jenny said 'Dog'; we then began to play with the ball as a dog. There was lots of laughter when the 'dog' ran away, and we took turns to retrieve the 'dog' and 'tell him off'. Jenny wanted to repeat this many times, in this and in the following session. (Therapist's clinical notes, Session 5)

It seemed that Jenny's one-to-one relationships became based on particular activities which were important for her to repeat, e.g. 'relaxing with Diane', and the 'dog game with Lynn'. Trevarthen *et al.* (1998) note that in autism there is a need to guard against rituals becoming stereotypical habits. Jenny tended towards habit formation, and Lynn and Diane needed to take care to vary the activities and help Jenny develop a variety of ways of relating. The use of different objects (in this case the use of the ball) offered an opportunity to Jenny to relate with another person in ways that guarded against the formation of stereotypical habits. It also enabled Jenny to move her way of relating beyond the sensory experience to the beginning of symbolic work and symbolic communication. This appeared to take place through Jenny sharing with Lynn her frustration for the absent member of the group in a playful manner (i.e. 'telling the dog off' for 'running away')

One-to-one relationship with Tim

Building relationships through embodiment play – 'I got you'

Tim's relationship with the therapist also started with what Jennings (1990, 1993, 1999, 2006) refers to as 'embodiment play'. It also had features of what Sherborne (2001) calls the 'shared relationship'. Although Tim had turned down initial attempts from Lynn to involve him in 'caring' developmental movement activities, he appeared delighted with lively games that developed with him having more control in the interaction. For instance, in Session 1 Tim (aged 11) refused to sit facing Lynn, so she sat behind him, swaying. In the therapist's clinical notes the following description can be found.

> Tim was looking to the side and as I swayed I got the feeling Tim was looking at me. I increased the sway to look at Tim and he started to sway in the opposite direction, smiling and turning his face away. Our movements became big and we swayed in rhythm. Eventually I doubled to 'catch Tim out' and we came face-to-face and I exclaimed, 'I got you!' Tim buried his face in his hands and squealed with delight: 'No'. I continued to sway and Tim immediately swayed again in perfect rhythm with me. The sense of fun and connection between us felt immense. (Therapist's clinical notes, Session 1)

In this game eye contact, which was fleeting and limited, appeared to be bearable for Tim. As Evans and Dubowski (2001) state, reciprocal cueing, where each person looks for and responds to cues in the other, can be used by the therapist to begin to establish a relationship with the child.

In many ways this interaction typified the play that Janert (2000) suggests can encourage the child with autism to attend to the other person, motivated to find out what they have in mind. Janert (2000) stresses the value of games of this kind because they create uncertainty and curiosity and involve emotions in an atmosphere of friendly affection. Janert also acknowledges the value in making movement, sound and expressions bigger as a way of catching and holding a child's attention. 'Affect attunement' (Stern 1985) occurred naturally in the play as a response to shared pleasure. Janert describes this sort of interaction as leading to a dynamic web of interpersonal events always responding to each other. This resembles the 'betweenness' of people, a definition of relationship (Clarkson 1994).

Building relationships through embodiment play – 'shooting and chasing games'

This theme developed further in subsequent sessions, as Tim would pretend either to die or 'shoot' Lynn when they 'caught each other out'. As

Lynn lay still, Tim would excitedly creep up to her and place his hand on her, to see if she would 'come to life'. Lord (2000) notes that people with autism may need human contact but may find touch distressing, and this may be because contact is experienced as unpredictable or uncontrolled. In this game Tim could control the touch as Lynn responded to his lead. An example can be found in the following extract from the therapist's clinical notes:

> I suggested we sit back-to-back and we gradually took turns leaning on each other. For a while there was rhythm and trust, as Tim took my weight and gave me all of his, leaning back, and lifting his hips. (Therapist's clinical notes, Session 6)

Sherborne (2001) notes how children develop confidence in their partner and in themselves in what she called 'shared relationships'. Tim learned to trust Lynn and to trust himself. This enabled him to move to another developmental stage in which 'against' relationships were explored, as the following extract shows.

> Then, while I was leaning on Tim, he quickly moved away and I fell to the floor. Tim 'shot' me and straightened my body then hovered nearby waiting expectantly. I 'came to life' as a robot-like 'monster' and began to chase Tim, slowly at first as he ran away, then more quickly. Tim was laughing excitedly and calling, 'Look Diane'. I momentarily caught Tim but immediately sensed his panic or fear, so I let go and he 'killed' me, rubbed his hands and walked away to sit on the ball, triumphantly whistling *Thunderbirds*. (Therapist's clinical notes, Session 6)

Evans and Dubowski (2001) note the need to be aware of advance and retreat, and discuss how the client often retreats when the therapist advances.

In the chasing game described above, Tim had experimented with allowing another person to have control. Brown (2002) points out how difficult this can be for some children with autism. This was a big step for Tim and he seemed to enjoy the excitement of the chase. However, he needed eventually to defeat the monster, and regain control, which he did with relish. Janert (2000) writes that the 'pretend threat' attracts the child 'at a physical survival or gut level, engaging his attention, motivation and interest', which is fundamental for developing cognitive skills, building confidence and supporting the development of a strong ego (Sherborne 2001).

Building relationships through role – 'the ambulance'

Tim and Diane's interactions developed through the use of what Jennings (1990, 1993, 1999, 2006) refers to as 'role'. For children to engage in role, an ability to symbolize is essential. Contrary to the common belief that children with autism cannot symbolize, Tim seemed to be able to engage in symbolic play, as the following extract shows.

> Tim chose a ball which became a plane, Diane's beanbag was a helicopter. Diane crashed the helicopter and said it was on fire. Tim mimed the flames. Diane asked for rescue and Tim mimed rain and said, 'Put rain on.' Diane asked Tim, 'Where will you take me?' Tim made an ambulance noise and they travelled around the room, their arms outstretched, dipping and swaying in rhythm together. Tim began to hum the *Thunderbirds* tune. (Therapist's clinical notes, Session 4)

It is relevant that Tim's plane became a Thunderbird, one of Tim's repetitive themes. Baker, Koegel and Kern Koegel (1998) note an increase in affect and social interaction when children with autism share games (with peers) using the child's 'obsessive' interests. Tim, who so often played in his own world, had found a way to share his world with a partner, albeit an adult, and in so doing actively began to engage with his partner in symbolic play. Wieder and Greenspan (2003) describe how symbolic play can promote the sharing of ideas and feelings. This can become an important part of relationship building.

Being part of a group – Tim and Jenny

Building relationships through shared leadership – 'the stop–go game'

The group relationship developed through repeated, structured group activities and the client-led creative play that developed from them. These often took the form of rituals. Although these rituals were not immediately taken up by the children, they were seen as important ways of providing a sense of safety that was essential for relationship building (Chesner 1995 Jennings 1990, 1993; Noble 2001), and as such they were repeated in each session. For instance, in Session 1, at first Tim refused to join in the 'story of the circle' dance. The group waited patiently and eventually Tim joined the dance, turning his head away from the circle. By Session 6 Tim and Jenny would both take a turn at telling 'the story of the circle' as the group all held hands and danced together, smiling and giving each other eye contact. The following extract refers to another group interaction that encouraged the development of group relationships. It became known as the 'stop–go' game.

> Tim rolled back as he caught the big body ball. I copied him and suggested we all try this and a game developed with lots of giggling as we rolled over and threw the ball between our legs from lying down. After more passing, Jenny lay with her feet on the ball and we all joined her, padding the ball with our feet. Tim said 'Wait' and I asked him to tell us when to 'stop' and 'go'. We took turns to be the leader. At first Tim would interrupt when Jenny was leading. (Therapist's clinical notes, Session 2)

The 'stop–go' game was requested in every session after this, involving shared pleasure, giggling and co-operation as Tim learned to respond to Jenny's, as well as the adults', lead.

This game encouraged Jenny's and Tim's spontaneity and creativity, providing affirmation and a connection between their individual worlds and the people in the world outside (Alverez and Reid 1999). Jennings (1983) refers to the communal aspect of sharing in and with others' creativity and drama. In these activities Jenny and Tim shared pleasure as part of a group, which was a big development for them in the school context. The value of shared activities in developing socialization, awareness of others and a sense of togetherness and belonging are well documented (Turry and Marcus 2003).

CHANGES IN CLIENT BEHAVIOUR OUTSIDE SESSIONS

Towards the end of the six weeks, outside of sessions, Tim began to play chasing games with his classmates in the playground, and to join in group discussions and P.E. lessons. Jenny's mother reported that she felt dramatherapy had made Jenny more outgoing, as Jenny would spontaneously tell her family about 'drama'. This was particularly important, considering the fact that normally Jenny would not volunteer to speak about school. A member of staff reported that Jenny, who had rarely approached her in the past, asked her to play table tennis.

After a four-week break the group received a further five sessions of dramatherapy, in which the play was developed, and play with puppets and other objects was introduced. Following this, Tim's mother noted 'a big change in Tim over the last few months'. She said that previously Tim would not speak unless spoken to, but now he would approach family members to talk to them. Tim's teacher noted that Tim would share a computer with a partner – something he had previously refused to do – and that he was 'more group-orientated'. Three months later it appeared that Tim was continuing this new behaviour.

CONCLUSIONS

Returning to the questions guiding this study (were relationships built in this group, and if so, how was their development supported?), it seemed that a number of different relationships were formed that, broadly speaking, fell into two categories: (1) one-to-one relationships, and (2) group relationships. Given the severity of autistic features of the two children involved in this dramatherapy group, there was a tendency for more one-to-one than group relationships. Still, both types were present. Contrary to the emphasis placed in some of the previous literature on sensory stimuli and movement-based engagement as the main way of interacting with children with autism, in this case a number of relationships were built which moved beyond embodiment play to projective work, and in a few instances to role.

Difficulties in generalizing from a case study have already been acknowledged. Based on the significant events presented and discussed, the following are some tentative conclusions regarding the potential value of working with children with autism in dramatherapy.

1. It is possible that dramatherapy can offer opportunities to children with autism to explore relationships in a number of different ways. Embodiment play (Jennings 1990, 1993, 1999, 2006) is one first level of work that can be considered when working with children with autism. Embodiment activities can involve:

   (a) sensory-based work. e.g. Jenny's 'relaxing with Diane'. This type of play can support the development of 'caring relationships' (Sherborne 2001) that create a first sense of relatedness. It is important that sensory work is encouraged in a way that taps into the child's existing movement preferences and is sensitive to their tolerance of touch and proximity to others

   (b) reciprocal cuing and rhythm, or what Stern (1985) refers to as 'affective attunement' (elsewhere found as mirroring, empathetic reflection, etc.; see Chapter 10 by Wengrower on dance movement psychotherapy). These movement-based strategies support the development of 'shared relationships' (Sherborne 2001) that involve shared control and 'mutuality', e.g. 'row your boat' and Tim and Lynn's 'I got you' game. These relationships also have a direct link with building trust. However, such movement work needs to be done in a sensitive non-threatening way, e.g. some clients will require/prefer limited eye contact

(c) teasing games that may allow for 'against' relationships (Sherborne 2001), and require spontaneity and playfulness, e.g. Tim and Lynn's 'shooting and chasing games'. Control, which is a pertinent issue for children with autism, can become a relevant exploration involving letting go and regaining control. This type of game can ultimately support the development of confidence.

2. Projective techniques may support the development of relationships in ways that children with autism can find bearable. Objects can encapsulate features of this relationship and involve aspects of symbolic work, e.g. Jenny and Lynn's 'dog game'. Considered use can also offer opportunities for diverse experiences and for guarding against the development of stereotypical habits.

3. Group interactions can be supported by sharing leadership in such a way that members engage in turn-taking, have opportunities to be seen and to see others, and can have opportunities to be or not to be part of the group, e.g. 'the stop–go game'. The use of props can be a particularly useful way of relating with the group as a whole, even more so than when one-to-one interactions take place.

4. Role is an area that children with autism are seen as not readily able to engage with. However, this study has shown that, although movement work is particularly important, children with autism can engage in role-playing, and thus symbolic work, especially when the child's own worldview and preferred themes are used as the topic of the symbolic play – e.g. Tim and Diane's 'ambulance play'. Symbolic work and imagination with the particular client group will be further discussed in the following chapter by Fuyuko Takeda on art therapy, and on the whole it seems to deserve further clinical consideration and research.

Other important factors that can be considered when starting with work with children with autism are: the need for an appropriate setting free from overwhelming stimuli; attention to group composition; and careful consideration of the structure of the session in a way that balances ritual and risk. Opportunities not to take part, and to engage in one-to-one activities, are important in group dramatherapy. In this study the particular approach adopted was sensitive to the developmental needs of the children involved, paid attention to individual differences, and involved dramatherapeutic methods to entice and interest the clients, including movement, play, visual cues and limited reliance on language (Chesner 1995). Furthermore, the one-to-one play resembled early parent–child intersubjectivity; these interactions form the foundations for the building of relationships (Stern 1985; Trevarthen *et al.* 1998). Key aspects remain the emotionality of these interactions (Alvarez and Reid 1999; Alvarez *et al.* 1999).

Further work based on ideas coming from developmental psychologists and child psychotherapists can inform the work taking place within dramatherapy with this client group. Research into effective ways of working in dramatherapy with children with autism also needs further development. This work will have to take into account knowledge generated from other neighbouring disciplines (e.g. Gold, Voracek and Wigram 2004 in music therapy; Loman 1995 in dance movement psychotherapy), and at the same time acknowledge and celebrate the unique contribution that dramatherapy can make within special education.

REFERENCES

Alvarez, A. and Reid, S. (1999) *Autism and Personality. Findings from the Tavistock Autism Workshop.* London: Routledge.

Alvarez, A., Reid, S., and Hodges, S. (1999) 'Autism and play – the work of the Tavistock autism workshop.' *Child Language Teaching and Therapy 15*, 1, 53–64.

Alvin, J. (1978) *Music Therapy for the Autistic Child.* Oxford: Oxford University Press.

Ansdell, G. and Pavlicevic, M. (2001) *Beginning Research in the Arts Therapies. A Practical Guide.* Tyne and Wear: Athenaeum Press.

Baker, M.J., Koegel, R.L. and Kern Koegel, L. (1998) 'Increasing the social behaviours of young children with autism using their obsessive behaviours.' *Journal of the Association for Persons with Severe Handicaps 23*, 4, 300–308.

Blotzer, M.A. (1995) 'Gilbert. Lost in Time.' In M.A. Blotzer and R. Ruth (eds) *Sometimes You Just Want to Feel Human. Case Studies of Empowering Psychotherapy with People with Disabilities.* Baltimore, MD: Paul. H. Brookes.

Brigg, G. (1996) 'From the Imagination. Language Development through Drama.' In A. Kempe (ed.) *Drama Education and Special Needs.* Cheltenham: Stanley Thorne.

Bromfield, R. (1992) *Playing for Real. The World of a Child Therapist.* London: Penguin.

Brown, S. (2002) 'Hullo Object! I Destroyed You!' In L. Bunt and S. Hoskyns *The Handbook of Music Therapy*. London: Brunner–Routledge.

Carrette, J. (1992) 'Autism and dramatherapy.' *Dramatherapy, the Journal of the British Association of Dramatherapists 14*, 2, 17–20.

Cesaroni, L. and Garber, M. (1991) 'Exploring the experiences of autism through first-hand accounts.' *Journal of Autism and Developmental Disorders 21*, 303–313.

Chesner, A. (1995) *Dramatherapy for People with Learning Difficulties*. London: Jessica Kingsley Publishers.

Clarkson, P. (1994) 'The Psychotherapeutic Relationship.' In P. Clarkson and M. Pokorny (eds) *The Handbook of Psychotherapy*. London: Routledge.

Crimmens, P. (2006) *Drama Therapy and Storymaking in Special Education*. London and Philadelphia, PA: Jessica Kingsley Publishers.

Elliot, R. and Shapiro, D.A. (1992) 'Client and Therapist as Analysts of Significant Events.' In S. G. Toukmanian and D.L. Rennie (eds) *Psychotherapy Process Research. Paradigmatic and Narrative Approaches*. London: Sage.

Evans, K. and Dubowski, J. (2001) *Art Therapy with Children on the Autistic Spectrum. Beyond Words*. London: Jessica Kingsley Publishers.

Gold, C., Voracek, M. and Wigram, T. (2004) 'Effects of music therapy for children and adolescents with psychopathology: a meta-analysis.' *Journal of Child Psychology and Psychiatry 46*, 6, 1054–1063.

Greenspan, S.I. and Wieder, S. (1997) 'Developmental patterns and outcomes in infants and children with disorders in relating and communicating: a chart review of 200 cases of children with autistic spectrum diagnoses.' *Journal of Developmental and Learning Disorders, 1*, 87–141.

Grainger, R. (1999) *Researching the Arts Therapies. A Dramatherapist's Perspective*. London: Jessica Kingsley Publishers.

Hobson, R.P. (2007) 'Communicative depths: soundings from developmental psychopathology.' *Infant Behaviour and Development 30*, 267–277.

Janert, S. (2000) *Reaching the Young Autistic Child. Reclaiming Non-Autistic Potential through Communicative Strategies and Games*. London: Free Association Books.

Jennings, S. (1983) 'Models of practice in dramatherapy.' *Dramatherapy. The Journal of the British Association for Dramatherapists 7*, 1, 3–6.

Jennings, S. (1990) *Dramatherapy with Families, Groups and Individuals. Waiting in the Wings*. London: Jessica Kingsley Publishers.

Jennings, S. (1993) *Playtherapy with Children: a Practitioner's Guide*. Oxford: Blackwell Scientific Publications.

Jennings, S. (1999) *Introduction to Developmental Playtherapy*. London: Jessica Kingsley Publishers.

Jennings, S. (2006) *Creative Play with Children at Risk*. Milton Keynes: Speechmark.

Jones, P. (1984) 'Therapeutic storymaking and autism, in art therapy as psychotherapy in relation to the mentally handicapped.' *Proceedings of a Conference on Art Therapy and the Mentally Handicapped, at Hertfordshire College of Art and Design*, 114–123.

Jones, P. (1996) *Drama as Therapy, Theatre as Living*. London: Routledge.

Jones, P. (2007) *Drama as Therapy: Theory, Practice and Research*. (Second edition.) London: Routledge.

Jordan, R. (2003) 'Social play and autistic spectrum disorders: a perspective on theory, implications and educational approaches.' *Autism 7*, 4, 347–360.

Josefi, O. and Ryan, V. (2004) 'Non-directive play therapy for young children with autism: a case study.' *Clinical Child Psychology and Psychiatry 9*, 4, 533–551.

Kalish, B.I. (1968) 'Body movement therapy for autistic children: a description and discussion of basic concepts.' *Journal of the American Dance Therapy Association 1*, 1, 7–9.

Lindkvist, M. (1977) 'Drama and Movement with Autistic Children.' In G. Shattner and R. Courtney, *Drama in Therapy. Volume 1: Children.* New York: Drama Book Specialists.

Loman, S. (1995) 'The Case of Warren: A KMP Approach to Autism.' In F. Levy (ed.) *Dance and Other Expressive Art Therapies.* New York: Routledge.

Lord, S. (2000) 'Dance and Drama.' In S. Powell and R. Jordan, *Autism and Learning. A Guide to Good Practice.* London: David Fulton.

Miller, S. (2005) 'Developing friendship skills with children with pervasive developmental disorders: a case study.' *Dramatherapy. The Journal of the British Association of Dramatherapists 27*, 2, 11–16.

Mittledorf, W., Hendricks, S. and Landreth, G.L. (2001) 'Play Therapy with Autistic Children.' In G.L. Landreth (ed.) *Innovations in Play Therapy. Issues, Process and Special Populations.* Philadephia: Brunner–Routledge.

Noble, J. (2001) 'Art as an Instrument for Creating Social Reciprocity: Social Skills Group for Children with Autism.' In S. Riley (ed.) *Group Process Made Visible. Group Art Therapy.* East Sussex: Brunner–Routledge.

Parteli, L. (1995) 'Aesthetic listening: contributions of dance movement therapy to the psychic understanding of motor stereotypes and distortions in autism and psychosis in childhood and adolescence.' *Arts in Psychotherapy 22*, 3, 241–247.

Robarts, J. (1996) 'Music Therapy and Children with Autism.' In C. Trevarthen, K. Aitken, D. Papoudi, J. Robarts (eds) *Children with Autism – Diagnosis and Interventions to Meet their Needs.* London: Jessica Kingsley Publishers.

Schopler, E. and Olley, J.G. (1982) 'Comprehensive Educational Services for Autistic Children: the TEACCH model.' In C.R. Reynolds and T.R. Gutkin (eds) *Handbook of School Psychology.* New York: Wiley.

Sherborne, V. (2001) *Developmental Movement for Children.* London: Worth Publishing.

Stern, D. (1985) *The Interpersonal World of the Infant.* New York: Basic Books.

Trevarthen, C., Aitken, K., Papoudi, D. and Robarts, J. (1998) *Children with Autism. Diagnosis and Interventions to Meet Their Needs.* London: Jessica Kingsley Publishers.

Turry, A. and Marcus, D. (2003) 'Using the Nordoff– Robbins Approach to Music Therapy with Adults Diagnosed with Autism.' In D.J. Weiner and L. Oxford *Action Therapy with Families and Groups, Using Creative Arts Improvisation in Clinical Practice.* Washington, DC: American Psychological Association.

Vygotsky, L.S. (1978) *Mind in Society: the Development of Higher Psychological Processes.* (Transl. from 1932). Cambridge, MA: Harvard University Press.

Wethered, A.G. (1993) *Movement and Drama in Therapy. A Holistic Approach.* London: Jessica Kingsley Publishers.

Wieder, S. and Greenspan, S.I. (2003) 'Climbing the symbolic ladder in the DIR model through floor time/interactive play.' *Autism 7*, 4, 425–435.

Williams, D. (1996) *Autism. An Inside-out Approach.* London: Jessica Kingsley Publishers.

Woodward, A. (2004) 'Music therapy for autistic children and their families: a creative spectrum.' *British Journal of Music Therapy 18*, 1, 8–14.

Yin, R.K. (2003) *Case Study Research: Design and Methods.* Thousand Oaks, CA: Sage.

Chapter 12

The Capacity for Imagination

Implication for Working with Children with Autism in Art Therapy

Fuyuko Takeda

INTRODUCTION

Setting the scene

Art therapy has gradually raised its profile in education, and is gaining a place within educational settings in the UK (Karkou 1999). In recent years, in particular since the introduction of the National Service Frameworks (NSF) by the Department of Health in 2004, the school has extended its role as a place for teaching and learning, and has provided a wide range of services including therapeutic support. According to the British Association of Art Therapists, over 150 art therapists are registered with the subgroup Art Therapy in Education (ATE).

Autistic spectrum disorders (ASD) are now estimated to affect one in 100 children in the UK (National Autistic Society 2006). The unique characteristics of autism are addressed with special provision, often within special education. This study took place in special primary schools for children with moderate learning difficulties in England. Each school had a special unit for children with ASD with specialized teaching staff. In line with the other state special schools in the UK, TEACCH (Treatment and Education of Autistic and (Related) Communication (Handicapped) CHildren) and PECS (Picture Exchange Communication Symbols) were employed in order for the pupils to access the National Curriculum.

This particular study grew out of my experience of working with children with autism since 2000. As an art therapist, I often come across children with autism who repeatedly draw certain characters from their favourite cartoons every week. It is also common that those children always produce their drawings in exactly the same order and use the same art materials. Other art therapists have also reported the rigidity in the artwork and behaviour, when working with children with autism (Evans 1998; Evans and Dubowski 2001; Meyerowitz-Katz 2008; Patterson 2008; Tipple 2003, 2008). I often wondered, however, whether or not their pictures could be interpreted in the same way as the ones made by children without autism, and about the degree to which imagination and imaginative work can be supported through art therapy.

The term 'imagination' is widely used in everyday life. In art therapy, therapists often use the term 'image' when referring to pictures made in art therapy sessions. Hillman (1960) argues that art therapy activates imagination and allows it to materialize. However, the area of imagination is known as one of the three main deficits in autism, alongside socialization and communication (Wing and Gould 1979). This chapter focuses primarily on children's capacity for imagination in art therapy and its implications for autism.

LITERATURE REVIEW

Autism and art therapy

The condition of autism was first described by Kanner in 1943. Until the mid-1980s, autism was generally believed to be caused by 'cold parenting' (Bettelheim 1967; Kanner 1943; Meltzer 1974; Tinbergen and Tinbergen 1983). However, autism is now considered to be caused by abnormal development of the brain (e.g. Castelli *et al.* 2002). Still, the existence of psychogenic autism (Tustin 1992) remains as an explanation supported by researchers and practitioners in psychoanalysis, as well as art therapists.

Evans (1998) provides one of the most important pieces of academic research on children with autism in the UK. She focuses on the development of communicative abilities and explores how the art-making process assists this development in children with autism. She challenges the existing psychodynamic object-relations approach that is often used in art therapy. Because of their specific communication difficulty, Evans (1998) argues that it is difficult to form a therapeutic relationship with children with autism. Instead, she applies early infant developmental theories, including development in drawing. A large part of her work is based on the developmental model proposed by Stern (1985), and she defines art therapy with children with autism as an alternative to psychotherapy – not as a form of psychotherapy (Evans 1998).

Imagination in cognitive psychology and psychodynamic psychotherapy

Imagination is defined and understood differently by different disciplines. Cognitive psychology has been one of the most influential fields in autism research for the last three decades. However, even within this field of study, research into the capacity for imagination in autism is far less common than other areas of impairments in autism: socialization and communication.

For example, the experiments conducted by Craig and Baron-Cohen (2000) used story-telling as a measure of investigation. They consider a story as 'imaginative' only when there are impossible or unreal elements within it. For example, if an elephant is walking in a forest, that is considered as non-imaginative, because it occurs in reality. On the other hand, if an elephant is talking with people, that would be seen as imaginative. The results from these experiments show that children with autism are less likely to use imaginative elements in their stories (Craig and Baron-Cohen 2000). Similarly, Scott and Baron-Cohen (1996) have reported that children with autism can understand the difference between what is possible and impossible, but cannot produce impossible pictures by themselves. Interestingly, Craig and Baron-Cohen (2000) fail to provide a definition of imagination in their study.

Conversely, within psychodynamic thinking, various attempts to define imagination have been made. For example, Winnicott (1971) notes a distinction between fantasy and imagination (the term 'dream' is used in the same context). He sees fantasy as a state of daydreaming, which can disturb a person's whole life. Fantasy does not have the capacity to be lived out in reality, nor can it relate to real objects. Neither does fantasy belong to playing, which is essential for creative living. He argues that there is no poetic value in fantasy; it is, in other words, a 'dead end'. Fantasy is operated within an isolated phenomenon, and it does not have connection with others. Therefore fantasy does not have a space where the psychotherapist can make an interpretation.

On the other hand, imagination (*dream*) is connected with others. Winnicott describes *dream* as 'formlessness', for example, like material before it is patterned, cut, shaped and put together. He also sees that dream has 'poetry in it'. Dream holds several different meanings that relate to past, present and future, and inner and outer. Dream fits into object-relating real worlds, where an interpretation can be made in psychotherapy (Winnicott 1971). While such definitions and models form the discipline of psychoanalysis and are useful in suggesting psychotherapeutic interventions, especially those based on interpretation, such definitions are of little use in helping us to understand the deficits of imagination in autism and, more particularly, the consequences of the deficit in respect to therapeutic practice and intervention with this client group. This state of ambiguity and potential confusion regarding what we mean by 'imagination' makes any research into the deficit of imagination in children (and adults) with autism very problematic. The following study highlights these problems and suggests some ways forward.

THE STUDY

Research question

Art therapy involves art-making, which is widely considered to be a very creative form of play. An understanding of the developmental process of the child is often considered important for art therapists working with children (Karkou and Sanderson 2006). For example, development can be understood as involving non-symbolic 'scribble' stages, 'named-scribble', and finally representation (Dubowski 1990). The question of whether exposure to art therapy gives rise to creativity and imagination underpins my research. More specifically, the research question for this study is as follows:

Can exposure to art therapy help in respect to the deficit of imagination associated with autism?

Design

The study involved a total of 12 children with autism from two special primary schools. The children were matched through the Test for Reception of Grammar (TROG) (Bishop 1983) and the Symbolic Play Test (Lowe and Costello 1976) before the study began. Half of the sample (the subject group; n = 6) received a 30-minute art therapy session on a weekly basis for the period of one academic year, and the remaining six children constituted the control group. The children in the control group did not receive any form of therapy, apart from speech and language therapy, during that period.

At a later stage, a case study design was considered as a better suited approach to the intervention and the data collected. The use of a case study is the most common form of a research design used by art therapists in the UK. Although it is described as lacking in 'representativeness' (Silverman 2005), it provides a depth of understanding of some particular phenomena that cannot be studied through quantitative methods. In this chapter I will concentrate primarily on findings from a boy with autism, whose case raises some interesting points for discussion regarding the use of art therapy for children with autism.

Methods of data collection

In this study, both quantitative and qualitative methods were employed. All 12 children (both the subject group and the control group) were tested on their play behaviours using Baron-Cohen's (1987) Pretend Play Test. The test encouraged play behaviour through different sets of toys and looked at these behaviours as falling under four types of play: sensorimotor, order, functional and pretend. It was chosen because there was no standard test to measure children's capacity for imagination *per se*; pretend play was seen as an aspect of imagination, and its absence as one of the criteria for predicting subsequent diagnosis of autism in young children aged 18 months (Baron-Cohen *et al.* 2000). Moreover, this test did not involve verbal interactions between the experimenter and the child, and so it was initially seen as more appropriate for this client group.

Children were assessed individually three times over the period of nine months, with intervals between the tests. For the children in both groups, the first test was carried out before the art therapy intervention started, and then the second test was conducted halfway through the study. Finally, at the end of the art therapy intervention, they took part in the last (third) test. Each child was videotaped individually in 18-minute segments, either in a self-contained room or in a corner of their classroom. A Chi square test was used to assess if there were any changes in the play behaviours between the two groups over the course of the study, while reflective notes kept from all sessions were analysed using thematic analysis.

Findings and discussion

QUANTITATIVE FINDINGS

Quantitative findings showed no significant difference in the abilities of the two groups in respect of pretend play (Chi square value = 0.074, df = 2, p >.05). Similarly, the other three stages of play categories did not show any changes between the subject and the control groups; sensorimotor (Chi square value = 0.364, df = 2, p >.05), ordered (Chi square value = 3.310, df = 2, p >.05), and functional play (Chi square value = 0.692, df=2, p >.05).

A number of reasons could explain these findings. First of all, the size of the sample was small, probably too small for any conclusive findings. Second, the timing of the data collection probably played a role. For example, the final play test was carried out during the last week of school term, when the school was busy and chaotic due to sports days and arrangements for trips. Similar to most children with autism, the children participating in this study found it difficult to cope with their routines being changed. As a consequence their ability to concentrate on the play test during this last week of the school year was limited. Moreover, the particular test also raised some questions as to the legitimacy of its assessment of their pretend play behaviours. For example, a child in the control group used the telephone as if he was speaking to someone, saying, 'Hello, Mrs Darcy, dinner is ready,' which is an act of pretending, according to the scoring criteria. However, he spoke in a monotonous voice throughout the test and also repeated the same phrases in his classroom, and so it was unclear to what extent he was 'pretending' during the test. It can be argued that the play test presented only a dimension of the capacity to pretend, and that the test result itself therefore did not explain all aspects of the capacity for imagination.

It is interesting that other forms of evidence contradict the quantitative findings. I will explore this further in the next section, in presenting a case study of the work completed in art therapy with Tom, a child with autism.

QUALITATIVE FINDINGS

Tom (pseudonym) was a ten-year-old with a diagnosis of autism and had been attending a special school since the age of six. His expressive language development was considerably delayed for his age group, but he could be seen as a child with moderate autism, as his receptive language and self-help skills were not severely impaired. According to his Special Educational Needs (SEN) statement, his language delay and lack of pretend play were particularly observed. His teachers informed me that he spoke little when he first came to the school. He had two older stepsisters and a younger sister. He lived with his mother, the second eldest stepsister, who was profoundly deaf, and the younger sister. He was on the Child Protection Register because he was suspected of having been sexually abused by his father when he was younger.

In many respects Tom presented as a typical child with autism at school. During my observation in the break time, he ran around in the playground endlessly and did not interact with other children at all. According to the staff, he used to take off all his clothes and run in the playground, even in the middle of winter. In the classroom, he played with Lego blocks by himself for a long time. He repeatedly piled up the blocks and brought his face very close to them, which was familiar behaviour in children with autism. From a play test perspective (Baron-Cohen 1987), his use of Lego blocks could be categorized as ordered play, not pretend play.

Art therapy sessions were held for 30 minutes on Mondays during the school terms. Tom attended 17 sessions in all and always had a rigid routine in each session. First, he took his shoes off when he came into the room. His sessions then normally consisted of three sections:

1. the whiteboard section: he always started by drawing on the whiteboard for approximately five minutes and changed his school T-shirt to the 'painting' T-shirt
2. the painting/pen section: he would then move to painting, sometimes making a drawing with a pen for 5–10 minutes
3. water/3D: then he would play with water and often made a 3D object.

Finally we would colour in a circle on the art therapy timetable. He would change his T-shirt again and leave the room. He never changed this sequence from the first session to the very last session.

In the first session, when I introduced our new timetable, Tom looked at the timetable on the wall, which he had used with the previous art therapist. After drawing on the whiteboard and some paintings, he put the plug in the sink and filled it with water nearly to the top of the sink. As he left the room, he looked at the timetable on the wall and said, 'No next Friday, another Friday, another Friday...' His sessions with the other art therapist had been on Fridays, while our sessions were on Mondays. I said, 'Tom, see you next Monday.' I felt that in this first session it was as if he showed me what he had done in the past. I also felt his strong resistance towards me. He made very little eye contact during the session. Similarly, at the end of the second session, he said, 'Friday, another Friday...' When I asked him what day today was, he said, 'Monday'. From this interaction, it seemed to me that he could 'imagine' how I might feel or think when he said 'Friday'. It was as if he wanted to inform me of his disappointment and did not want to finish with the previous art therapist.

In the fifth session, after the Christmas break, he asked me to help him make a boat with a piece of paper and sticky tape. He filled the sink with water as usual and floated the boat on the water. However, the boat had gaps between the sticky tapes and sank after a while. He said, 'Boat is sinking, boat is sinking...' The time was nearly at an end and I suggested we should finish. He was very unhappy about finishing on that day. I said to him that we could make another boat the following week. I felt that a certain degree of therapeutic relationship had been formed between us at this stage. It seemed that by this time he could tolerate the change of therapist, and he did not say 'Friday' any more. The whole art therapy process became more co-operative without having much verbal communication. In that particular session, for example, our movement, the sound of water, and our interaction in making the same object felt smooth and comfortable.

The following week, Tom asked me to make a boat again. I stuck sticky tape more carefully than the previous week so as not to make a hole, because I did not want the boat to sink again. 'We' had a strong feeling of wanting to succeed, which seemed to be a phenomenon of intersubjectivity (Stern 1985). He then took more than ten coloured pencils and put them on the boat, and floated it on the water. However, the paper was very thin and absorbed water quickly. He said, 'Sinking, I'm sinking'. He seemed to be upset and made a hole in the boat with a finger, and finally crumpled it up. He then suddenly took all the papers out of the sand tray that was used as a paper tray on the floor. He placed the tray slantwise to the sink, and he turned on the tap. The water went onto the tray and dripped into the sink. He said, 'Waterfall' (see Figure 12.1). It was completely unpredictable. None of the children had ever used the sand tray the way he used it. While the water was running, I was afraid that it could overflow. However, I decided to leave him until the water reached the top of the sink. In fact the water did not overflow, and he controlled the tap precisely. When he left the room, he said, 'Thank you'.

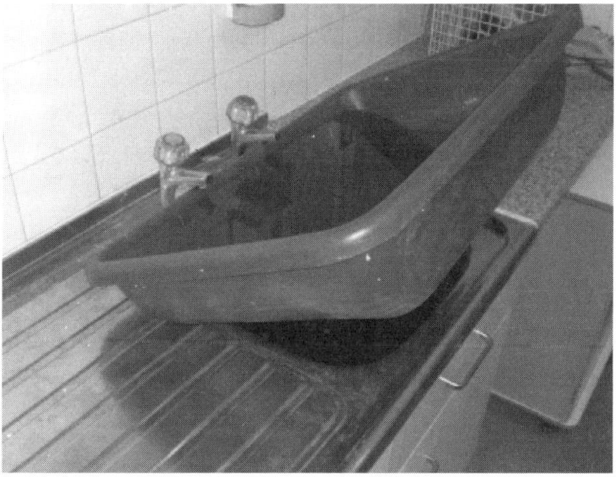

Figure 12.1: The waterfall (Session 6)

In the next session, he gave me a piece of paper and said 'submarine'. He folded the paper and made a cone, and asked me to put on the sticky tape. We also made two circles and stuck them onto the side of the cone. He then cut a small piece of the paper and made a pole. He seemed to be satisfied with the shape of the submarine and put it in the water. He said again, 'Look, sinking, I'm sinking.' I asked if he was in the submarine. He said, 'Yes'. I said that a submarine was made for under the sea and it was safe inside. He did not say anything and crumpled it up (Figure 12.2). I wondered if my interpretation was unsatisfactory for him.

He made a 'paper bridge' (Figure 12.3) in a later session. He wanted me to help him put the bridge over the sink. He then started to use brushes, which he pretended were people crossing the bridge. He pushed them strongly, so the bridge broke. I suggested that we could repair it together. He cut a small piece of paper and added it to the middle of the bridge. In the next few weeks, he made similar bridges. He always said, 'We need a bridge,' and used brushes as if they were walking on the bridge. During this period, he made a hole in his bridge with brushes and said, 'Look, the bridge is falling,' and also said, 'Look, I am sinking.' I replied, 'Maybe you can swim.' He then pretended to 'swim' with the brushes and cross the bridge.

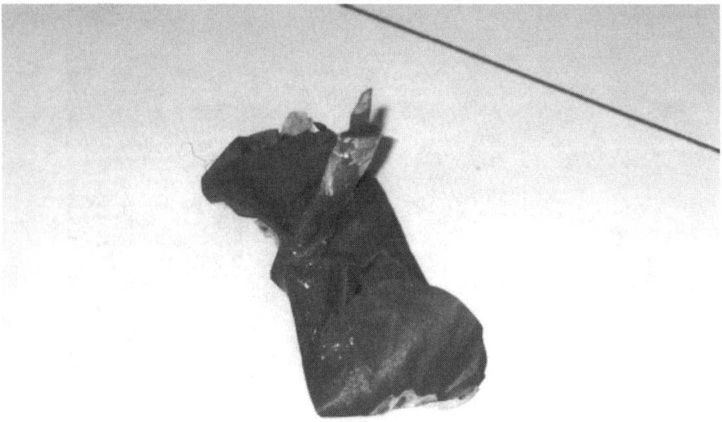

Figure 12.2: The submarine (Session 7)

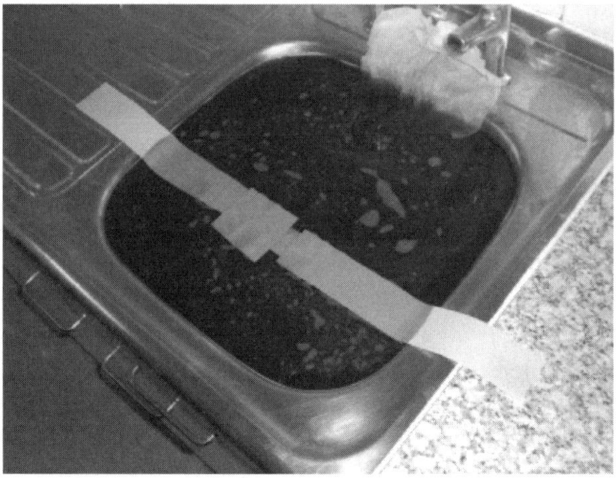

Figure 12.3: Paper bridge (Session 11)

He often made red water in the sink towards the end of the programme, which reminded me of blood. I did not instantly make interpretations, but I remembered that it was suspected that he had been sexually abused by his father in a bathroom. When I asked him if red water was clean or dirty water, he said, 'Dirty water'. If red water was associated with the traumatic experience, it would appear to be important for him to control the water by creating objects such as boats and bridges.

In the very last session, he made a drawing with many circles (Figure 12.4) resembling our timetable (Figure 12.5). Whilst he was drawing the circles, he said 'You see, Monday, Monday, Monday…many Mondays…' He then wrote his initial on the top left corner and coloured in the first circle. He hid our timetable under the art materials tray and said, 'You see, this is a new timetable.' By making his new timetable, it seemed to me, he was telling me that his art therapy was not long enough, and he wanted to continue.

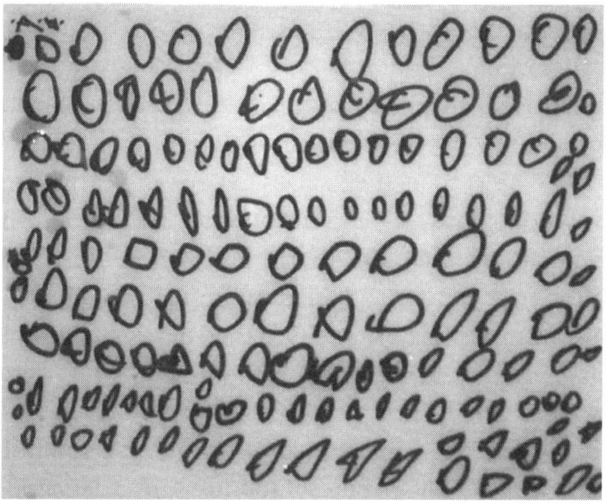

Figure 12.4: Drawing of timetable by Tom (last session)

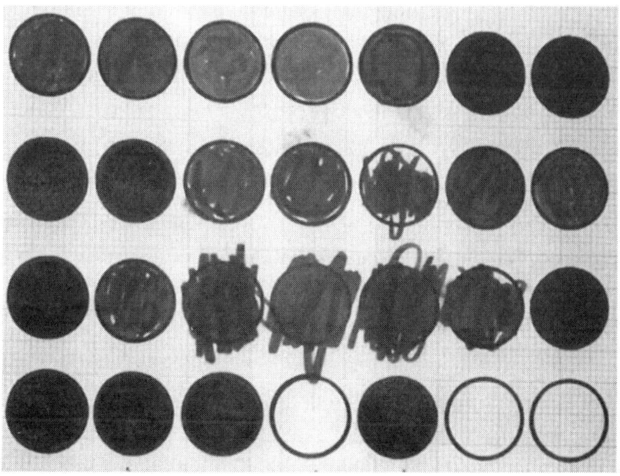

Figure 12.5: Original timetable for art therapy

Discussion

The general notion is that children with autism do not have the capacity for imagination, but the case of Tom presented a challenge that contradicted this notion. He demonstrated the capacity for imagination in his use of artwork and in his behaviours in the art therapy sessions.

It seems important to refer back to the definition of imagination as discussed amongst cognitive psychologists and psychoanalysts. For example, boats or bridges might not be regarded as imaginative from a cognitive psychology perspective, because they can exist in reality. However, there was a narrative structure in all of Tom's sessions. All of his objects had the legitimate quality of imagination as defined by Winnicott (1971). They did not remain as an isolated phenomenon, but were able to be shared with me. They related to the past, present and future, and inner and outer, while still remaining as objects in themselves. Tom set a structure by himself (whiteboard, painting/drawing and 3D/water), and within this framework he was 'freeing his imagination' through all his sensory aspects. Every element of water, such as sound, temperature, smell and touch, was present in the sessions. My role was to facilitate the environment where he could feel safe to play with water.

What Tom had tried during art therapy was to control the water in the sink, which may have contained unconscious, symbolic contents. Whether or not the red water represented his early traumatic experiences is uncertain. However, he used water as the main focus of his art therapy sessions. He said 'I'm sinking' when he used pens or brushes, and also made a brush 'swim' in the water. While in the classroom he just piled up Lego blocks, in art therapy he showed his capacity to pretend.

Knill (1998) suggests that the sensory aspects of imagination are important, which means that we often imagine sounds, rhythms, movements, and so on, as well as pictures. It seems that imagination as defined by cognitive psychology requires higher cognitive ability; but the more instinctive element of imagination does not. Sensory aspects of imagination are not visible and cannot be estimated in experiments. With Tom, the sensation from the water might have been a vehicle to encourage his capacity to pretend, in the context of art therapy in the presence of an art therapist.

CONCLUSION

In this chapter I have discussed art therapy with children with autism, focusing on the capacity for imagination. The quantitative findings provided no strong evidence to suggest that exposure to art therapy makes significant improvements in respect of the capacity for imagination in children with autism. However, I have also presented the case of a child with autism who seemed to have improved this capacity during the course of art therapy. It is important to emphasize again that Tom was a typical boy with autism in the school. He avoided eye contact and exhibited, on the face of it, a very rigid and repetitive pattern of behaviour. However, as the therapy unfolded, he increasingly exhibited his capacity for imaginative work and I became more and more aware of the unconscious symbolic content of his artwork and his behaviour.

I would not argue that the capacity for imagination is created from 'nothing' through art therapy. The severity of autism may well determine the extent of the capacity for imagination. I can only hypothesize that art therapy can offer a more primitive form of experience in promoting imagination for some children with autism, which might later be developed into a cognitive capacity for imagination. This study has shown contradictions in the existing knowledge about autism. It has also highlighted the complexity of the condition and raised important questions for art therapists working with these children. As such it raises as many questions as it presents answers. However, it is through the process of asking such questions that we can develop this discipline further.

REFERENCES

Baron-Cohen, S. (1987) 'Autism and symbolic play.' *British Journal of Developmental Psychology 5*, 139–148.

Baron-Cohen, S., Wheelright, S., Cox, A., Baird, G., Charman, T., Swettenham, J., Drew, A. and Doehring, H. (2000) 'Early identification of autism by the CHecklist for Autism in Toddlers (CHAT).' *Journal of the Royal Society of Medicine 93*, 521–525.

Bettelheim, B. (1967) *The Empty Fortress: Infantile Autism and the Birth of the Self.* USA: Free Press.

Bishop, D. (1983) *The Test for Reception of Grammar.* Published by the author and available from: Age and Cognitive Performance Research Centre, University of Manchester, M13 9PL.

Castelli, F., Frith, C.D., Happé, F. and Frith, U. (2002). 'Autism, Asperger Syndrome and brain mechanisms for the attribution of mental states to animated shapes.' *Brain 125*, 1839–1849.

Craig, F. and Baron-Cohen, S. (2000) 'Story-telling ability in children with autism or Asperger Syndrome: a window into the imagination.' *Israel Journal of Psychiatry and Related Sciences 37*, 64–70.

Dubowski, J. (1990) 'Art versus language: separate development during childhood.' In C. Case and T. Dalley (eds) *Working with Children in Art Therapy*. London: Routledge.

Evans, K. (1998) 'Shaping experience and shaping meaning.' *Inscape 3*, 17–25.

Evans, K. and Dubowski, J. (2001) *Art Therapy with Children on the Autistic Spectrum*. London: Jessica Kingsley Publishers.

Hillman, J. (1960) *Emotion*. Chicago, IL: NW University Press.

Kanner, L. (1943) 'Autistic disturbances of affective contact.' *Nervous Child 2*, 217–250.

Karkou, V. (1999) 'Art therapy in education: findings from a nationwide survey in arts therapies.' *Inscape 4*, 2, 62–70.

Karkou, V. and Sanderson, P. (2006) *Arts Therapies: A Research-based Map of the Field*. Great Britain: Elsevier Churchill Livingstone.

Knill, P.J. (1998) 'Soul Nourishment, or the Intermodal Language of Imagination.' In S.K. Levine and E.G. Levine (eds) *Foundation of Expressive Arts Therapy: Theoretical and Clinical Perspectives*. London and Philadelphia, PA: Jessica Kingsley Publishers.

Lowe, M. and Costello, A. (1976) *Symbolic Play Test*. Windsor: The NFER-Nelson Publishing Company Ltd.

Meltzer, D. (1974) 'Mutism in infantile autism, schizophrenia and manic-depressive states: the correlation of clinical psychopathology and linguistics.' *International Journal of Psycho-Analysis 55*, 397–404.

Meyerowitz-Katz, J. (2008) 'Other People Have a Secret that I Do Not Know: Art Psychotherapy in Private Practice with an Adolescent Girl with Asperger's Syndrome.' In C. Case and T. Dalley (eds) *Art Therapy with Children*. London: Routledge.

National Autistic Society (2006) *What is Autism?* London: The National Autistic Society.

Patterson, Z. (2008) 'From "Beanie" to "Boy."' In C. Case and T. Dalley (eds) *Art Therapy with Children*. London: Routledge.

Scott, F. and Baron-Cohen, S. (1996) 'Imagining real and unreal things: evidence of a disassociation in autism.' *Journal of Cognitive Neuroscience 8*, 371–382.

Silverman, D. (2005) *Doing Qualitative Research*. (Second edition.) London: Sage Publications.

Stern, D.N. (1985) *The Interpersonal World of the Infant*. London: Karnac Books.

Tinbergen, N. and Tinbergen, E.A. (1983) *Autistic Children: New Hope for a Cure*. UK: George Allen & Unwin Ltd.

Tipple, R. (2003) 'The interpretation of children's art work in a paediatric disability setting.' *Inscape,* 8, 48–59.

Tipple, R. (2008) 'Paranoia and Paracosms: Brief Art Therapy with a Youngster with Asperger's Syndrome.' In C. Case and T. Dalley (eds) *Art Therapy with Children*. London: Routledge.

Tustin, F. (1992) *Autistic States in Children*. (Revised edition.) London/New York: Routledge.

Wing, L. and Gould, J. (1979) 'Severe impairments of social interaction and associated abnormalities in children: epidemiology and classification.' *Journal of Autism and Developmental Disorders 9*, 11–29.

Winnicott, D.W. (1971) *Playing and Reality*. London: Routledge.

Chapter 13

Music Therapy for Children with Autism in an Educational Context

Jo Tomlinson

INTRODUCTION

Setting the scene

I have been working as a music therapist in special needs schools in the UK since 1995 primarily working with children on the autistic spectrum. I am employed by the local county music service, Cambridgeshire Music, which currently has a well established team of ten music therapists working in mainstream and special needs schools. I shall reflect on aspects of autism and how music may be used as a therapeutic intervention, and then go on to describe a case study of music therapy with a five-year-old boy with autism, within a school setting.

LITERATURE REVIEW

Autistic spectrum disorders are different from other types of disability in their social and emotional components (Asperger 1944; Frith 1989; Kanner 1943; Wing 1991). Many causes for autism have been speculated over the last 50 years, often apportioning blame to vulnerable families (Bettelheim 1967). The general opinion now is that autism is caused by neurological or biological factors, and brain scans can reveal abnormalities which create autistic 'charateristics'.

Autism is a particularly difficult disability for parents to come to terms with. In Baron-Cohen and Bolton (1993) a mother describes the emotional pain of dealing with her son's autistic behaviour: 'The more difficult his behaviour became, the more convinced I was that he was just doing it to spite me – to shut me out, to break my will, to win. I desperately wanted him to share in my world, but try as I might, everything was always on his terms' (p.26).

Music therapy can be extremely effective in creating opportunities for children with autism to expand and nurture their expressive and social skills. The National Autistic Society website (section on music therapy) states that: 'Music therapy has become accepted as a useful intervention for people with autism since it was introduced in the 1950s and 60s by practitioners like Juliette Alvin, Paul Nordoff and Clive Robbins'. More recently literature on music therapy and autism in the UK has expanded, and this has included research that provides evidence that this intervention is effective (Brown 1994; Bunt and Hoskyns 2002; Edgerton 1994; Howat 1995; Levinge 1990; Oldfield 2006; Patey-Tyler 2003; Robarts 1996, 1998; Warwick and Alvin 1978, Wigram 2002, Woodward 2003, 2004).

The approach to helping and teaching children with autism is much debated and discussed within the school context; this tends to be based on the level of structure and organization the child receives in the classroom and to what extent they are protected from the unpredictability of everyday life. Some approaches provide the child with an extremely structured and routine environment, so that they can then focus on fulfilling 'academic' tasks. For example, the Treatment and Education of Autistic and related Communication-handicapped CHildren (TEACCH) method is based on the theory that 'children with autism benefit more from a structured educational environment than from free approaches' (National Autistic Society website section on TEACCH).

Other approaches provide a certain amount of structure, but then also allow the child to experience a less controlled and predictable environment, i.e. a more life-like environment that is not so geared to the demands and obsessive tendencies of children with autism.

The type of environment the child experiences in the classroom may well have an impact on the way he or she responds to the music therapy environment. Sometimes I replicate elements of structure that are provided in the class setting, as this is the only way that the child can feel secure and able to establish a constructive relationship with me; alternatively I may feel a need to provide a freer, more relaxed approach, so as to allow the child to explore the music therapy environment in a way that would not be possible in the class context. My communication with staff at the school and with the child's parents is imperative in informing my decision about what type of approach to take.

I shall now move on to my case study; this illustrates the way in which I alternated between imposing structure and allowing space for exploration in my work with Oliver (name changed to ensure confidentiality), a boy with autism.

THE STUDY

Aim

This study aimed to explore the process of using music therapy with a child with autism within a special needs school.

Methodology

Given the exploratory aim, a case study design was selected as the most appropriate research strategy. Case studies, according to Yin (2003), allow investigation of complex social phenomena in real-life contexts. The art therapist Edwards (1999) suggests that the value of a case study is that it is 'personal' and attaches importance to individuality and subjective human experience.

The material collected for this study was 'naturally occurring' (Ansdell and Pavlicevic 2001) and reflected the process and development of the music therapy work. Clinical notes written after each session and video recordings were used as a record of the process and musical developments.

In this study I immersed myself in the material, formulating main themes and also reflecting on literature reviewed (Meekums 1993). In choosing this method of analysis I have attempted to present a set of predominant themes, retaining the narrative quality inherent in the work. Description of these themes and interpretation of their meaning are key features of the study. This type of analysis can be linked with hermeneutic phenomenology (Laverty 2003; McLeod 2001), where the researcher's 'fore-understanding' and culture impact on the way the material is reviewed. In this way I shall be presenting ideas based on my training and experiences, making reference to music therapy literature.

Findings and discussion

INTRODUCING OLIVER

Oliver is a child with whom I worked for two years at his special needs school. He had a diagnosis of autism and was five years old when I started working with him. The class Oliver was in used the structured TEACCH method; he was just beginning to adjust to the routines within this system when I commenced music therapy.

Oliver was frequently resistant to intervention or direction and sometimes found contact with other people difficult to tolerate. However, he would periodically show signs of great affection and would sometimes rush up to people and cuddle them. This had to be on his terms, and he tended to retreat irritably if he felt out of control of the interaction. Oliver's need to control his environment often led him to react aggressively and express rage if he felt that other people were not conforming to his demands. These reactions often took the form of screaming, shouting, or throwing things round the room, or sometimes hitting out at people. Oliver would happily explore objects and, if left on his own, could amuse himself independently for a certain period of time. At times he would become attention-seeking and restless when bored with an activity.

Throughout my work with Oliver I was in communication with his class teacher and his learning support assistant, so that I could feed back to them about his progress in music therapy and they could inform me of any developments in the class setting. I also met on a termly basis with Oliver's mother to share information and show video extracts of our work together.

INITIAL MEETING

Oliver came in to the room willingly but was not able to sit still for the 'hello song'. He dashed from one instrument to another, often running to get to an instrument and then moving on before I could engage him in any sort of interactive play. We had some fleeting moments of shared, focused play at the piano, when Oliver explored moving up and down the piano keys. He also showed delight and interest when I suddenly played my flute, but this was short-lived and he soon became restless again.

Oliver's playing on the instruments came in bursts and expressed frustration and agitation. He would suddenly make a dash for the drum, making growling vocal sounds and banging loudly and frenetically on the instrument. As soon as I attempted to join him in the playing he would run off again. Oliver could not sit still for the 'goodbye song' either, and we finished the session after about 15 minutes, as his concentration was deteriorating further.

It was quite difficult to feel positive about this first session, as it had been very fragmented with little interactive play. However, there were several factors that made me conclude that Oliver could benefit from further music therapy input. First, Oliver's fleeting but spontaneous reaction to my flute playing; he was able to look up and sustain eye contact while I played my flute. Although this was a momentary response it felt very positive. Oliver's fascination with the musical instruments for short periods of time, and his concentration whilst exploring them, encouraged me to feel that this was something which could be developed. In addition to this, Oliver vocalized expressively. This at times appeared to be communicative, and I felt that these sounds could be developed and supported through interactive music-making. Last, Oliver had the ability to play in outbursts of seemingly cathartic playing. Although these were very fragmented and non-interactive I felt hopeful that this type of playing could be extended, and that it might help Oliver to express some of his frustration constructively.

FIRST SIX MONTHS OF THERAPY: INDEPENDENT EXPLORATION

During this period Oliver often avoided any form of contact or interaction with me by moving rapidly from one activity to another. He would show fleeting moments of interest in the drum or xylophone, move over to them and explore them for a while, but then retreat as soon as I came over to join him. Often, if I left him to explore the instruments independently, he would become destructive with them, so that I would have to intervene. Generally my intervention would evoke rage and frustration in Oliver. He would then run around screaming and shouting, trying to destroy any instrument in his path. This sometimes involved pushing the large drum over with full force.

In calmer periods of exploration Oliver took the xylophone apart and lined up the bars on the floor, tapping each one in turn with the beater. He disliked being disturbed during this activity and pushed my hands away if I tried to join in.

Alvin and Warwick (1991) break down the music therapy process with children with autism into different stages of development. The first stage involves much independent exploration of the musical instruments, as 'autistic children can relate to objects better than to persons...the manipulation of this musical object is usually a source of great pleasure to the autistic child... It is beneficial because of the perceptual and motor control processes involved' (Alvin and Warwick 1991, p.13).

In the further stages they describe how the child develops a sense of trust in the therapist who accepts this initial exploratory behaviour. Gradually the therapist contributes more, both musically and verbally, to support the child's exploration, at which point 'the child should develop a sense of musical, social behaviour towards his instruments and the use of his voice...his need for self-expression, his relationship with [me], and the demands made by music itself...' (Alvin and Warwick 1991, p.23).

Oliver did enjoy playing up and down the piano keys, allowing me to sit with him while he did this, as long as I didn't try to intervene. He also occasionally joined me in strumming the autoharp, although his concentration during this activity was limited.

Throughout this period Oliver seemed to have a strong desire to keep himself separate from me and to avoid any form of direct interaction. If at any point Oliver felt out of control of the situation, his response would be to express his agitation through aggression towards the instruments, or occasionally me. There was little obvious change or development in therapeutic terms, although Oliver still continued to show fragmentary interest in the music. Oliver's displays of rage were confusing, as they did not seem to occur in response to any consistent context.

DIRECTIVE AND NON-DIRECTIVE INTERVENTIONS

Oliver's rejection of my involvement in his exploration of the instruments expressed a need to be independent. At the same time much of his behaviour was demanding and attention-seeking. His need to control had led him to develop certain strategies and patterns of interaction through which to do this. I attempted two ways of responding to Oliver's avoidant and destructive behaviour. First, I tried being more directive with Oliver, giving the sessions a clearer structure and trying to encourage interactive playing. This approach caused him to react with more avoidant responses, as he could not cope with losing his sense of control. Second, I allowed Oliver more space and freedom to explore the instruments and encouraged him to approach me, by being non-intrusive and absorbed into my own playing. This initially caused Oliver to become increasingly attention-seeking and difficult, but over time drew his attention into what I was doing.

Amelia Oldfield (1995) discusses this balance between following and initiating when working with children, and the decision of the therapist to work in a directive or non-directive way at different points in a session: 'the correct balance between directive and non-directive work can be used towards therapeutic ends by the music therapist' (p.237).

In between the difficulties with Oliver there were moments of sustained eye contact and interactive playing, which made me feel that he would be able to develop his interest in the music and build a more positive relationship with me. His ability to periodically explore the instruments with focused concentration and involvement also felt extremely constructive. My flute playing was something that immediately caught Oliver's attention and he would look up at me and sometimes smile in response to this. In each session he generally only responded once in this way and would then lose interest, so that it did not enable me to engage him in any form of interactive playing.

Oliver's vocalizing could be extremely expressive and this was something he used periodically in order to communicate feelings of frustration. His agitated vocalizing usually consisted of 'eee' sounds or 'na-na-na' if I was encouraging him to do something he didn't want to do, or if I tried to prevent him being destructive with the instruments. The frustration seemed to be partly a result of being unable to express verbally how he felt. The very positive aspect of his vocalizing was that it always felt communicative rather than self-absorbed, and expressed a desire for me to know how he was feeling. He would also say 'ba ba' when I said goodbye to him at the ends of sessions.

SECOND HALF OF TREATMENT: DEVELOPMENT OF INTERACTIVE PLAY

During this period of therapy Oliver gradually began to respond to the security and consistency of the sessions and became able to focus for increased periods of time on interactive as well as independent, exploratory music-making. I had put certain limitations on the number of musical instruments available to Oliver in the previous block of sessions, and now I put further restrictions on these. This seemed to make the sessions less chaotic and I selected specific instruments that Oliver was able to play more constructively. These were the piano, autoharp, drum and flute. We managed to establish various interactive games with which Oliver could feel familiar and confident. Instead of chasing after him when he ran round the room, I actually initiated running around as soon as I had sung the 'hello song' to Oliver. He smiled and laughed spontaneously in response to this and began running round after me. This became a regular activity which we did after periods of focused playing, and seemed to serve as a release of energy for Oliver.

Oliver also established a peek-a-boo game while I was playing the 'hello song', hiding behind the piano and looking out periodically to have eye contact with me. He occasionally smiled if I shouted 'Boo!' in response to this. This exchange created a positive sharing experience which replaced his resistance to sitting down for the 'hello song'.

David Cohen (1993) discusses the importance of play and 'peek-a-boo' games and how essential it is for children to experience this type of exchange in order to understand basic human concepts of communication. Cohen (1993) suggests: 'By being socialized into the game, the child is socialized into many basic exchanges of life' (p.104).

During this phase of therapy the nature of our interactive playing completely changed. Oliver began to be able to sit opposite me, sharing the autoharp, and carefully and independently strummed across the strings, focusing extremely intently on the sound he was producing. He was able to take turns during this activity and seemed to enjoy listening to my playing and anticipating his turn to play.

Oliver developed an interest in the ocean drum and was also able to share in playing this with me. We took it in turns, banging loudly on the drum, and then Oliver would slowly allow the beads to roll around the drum, watching them with fascination.

Oliver's interest in the flute also developed and his momentary responses to my playing became more sustained. He began to point at the flute to encourage me to play it and then smiled in response to the sound.

Oliver's vocal sounds developed and became increasingly communicative. At times the pitch of his vocalizing tuned in to the sound of the autoharp, particularly if I was singing along to this. We were able to share in some imitative vocalization and Oliver seemed more aware of me copying his vocal sounds.

As Oliver's playing became more interactive it also became more freely expressive and he was able to direct some of the energy that he had been putting into being destructive with the instruments into constructive playing. Sometimes there was an overlap between the two and Oliver would be playing loudly and cathartically on the ocean drum and then suddenly throw it on the floor. On the whole, though, his approach to the playing became far more focused and controlled, with a new awareness of expressive playing.

At this stage it seemed that Oliver's perception of my involvement in the session changed from that of a directive adult trying to prevent him from doing things, to someone who was interested in becoming involved in activities he had initiated. My running around possibly prevented him from continuing with his old pattern of destructive use of the instruments, and my involvement in this appealed to Oliver's sense of humour and consequently made him want to join in with the activity.

Towards the end of our work together I discussed Oliver's development in the music therapy sessions with his mother, who mentioned that he responded enthusiastically to several songs: 'Jingle bells', 'Five little ducks went swimming one day' and 'Postman Pat'. I decided to play these in the session and see what Oliver's response to them was. I sang the 'hello song' as usual, after which Oliver began moving around the room. Almost immediately afterwards I started to play 'Jingle bells'. Oliver's face became transfixed and he listened intently to my singing. After the song had finished I began singing it again, this time stopping before the last word in each phrase. Oliver carefully whispered the last word in each phrase. This was the first time I had heard Oliver form and produce words and it was a very exciting moment. This level of sharing felt like a leap forward in terms of his ability to respond socially to me within the session. His use of eye contact while I played and sang the songs was more sustained and consistent than previously, and he was able to anticipate parts of the songs.

This interaction lasted for about five minutes and Oliver then returned to his usual pattern of behaviour, periodically listening as I interspersed his familiar songs throughout the session.

CONCLUSION

For Oliver, music therapy was a very effective form of treatment and helped him with many different aspects of his social and expressive abilities. Although it is difficult to generalize from this one case to the whole population of children with autism, in my experience of working with children in schools I have found that music therapy can be a constructive intervention for many. The dramatic changes presented and discussed here for Oliver constitute just one example of changes that have taken place with other children with similar difficulties. Additionally I have found patterns emerging in my work with the same client group in relation to providing space for exploration in the early stages, which is then replaced by increased structure and intensity of interaction in the later phase of therapy.

It is possible that, as discussed here in my work with Oliver, the contributing factors for therapeutic changes are related to the music providing a stimulus for gaining and sustaining attention and a means through which the therapist can engage the child in interactive play. Through this type of exchange, concentration levels in relation to shared activity may increase. The consistency and predictability of the sessions as part of the school timetable can enable the child to develop the ability to relax and concentrate for short periods of time within this framework. This secure structure can facilitate exploration of the environment and the relationship with the therapist. Within this medium the therapist can combine respect for the child's individuality, and expressive qualities, with attempting to provide motivation to overcome aspects of their disability through musical exchange.

Children with autism tend to have an innate desire to control, due to the anxieties associated with interactive exchange with other people, and as a result can sometimes become entrenched in repetitive behavioural patterns. However, once they are convinced of the pleasures and empowerment of meaningful interaction, they can often be guided towards acquiring social skills that most individuals take for granted.

Oliver enjoyed developing his use of vocal sounds in the sessions, and occasionally began to tune into the music with these. My imitation of Oliver's vocalizing helped him to become more aware of the communicative aspects of vocal exchanges. Familiar songs can provide children with a secure base through which to explore their developing understanding of verbal communication and interaction. They can also anticipate significant words and phrases in the context of songs.

Oliver began to develop his expressive playing and started to use this as a channel for feelings of rage and frustration, but also as a means of expressing the calmer side of his personality. It is possible that music therapy sessions can generally provide an opportunity for children with autism to express a whole range of emotions.

Further research is needed in order to achieve a deeper understanding of how the emotional and communicative needs of children with autism can be best addressed within music therapy in an educational context.

REFERENCES

Alvin, J. and Warwick, A. (1991) *Music Therapy for the Autistic Child.* Oxford: Oxford University Press.

Ansdell, G. and Pavlicevic, M. (2001) *Beginning Research in the Arts Therapies: A Practical Guide.* London: Jessica Kingsley Publishers.

Asperger, H. (1944) 'Die "aunstisehen Psychopathen" im Kindesalter.' *Archiv für Psychiatrie und Nervenkrankheiten 117,* 76–136.

Baron-Cohen, S. and Bolton, P. (1993) *Autism: The Facts.* (Fifth edition.) Oxford: Oxford University Press.

Bettelheim, B. (1967) *The Empty Fortress: Infantile Autism and the Birth of the Self.* New York: Free Press.

Brown, S. (1994) 'Autism and music therapy: is change possible and why music?' *British Journal of Music Therapy 8,* 1, 15–25.

Bunt, L. and Hoskyns, S. (2002) *The Handbook of Music Therapy.* London: Routledge.

Cohen, D. (1993) *The Development of Play.* (Second edition.) London: Routledge.

Edgerton, C. L. (1994) 'The effect of improvisational music therapy on the communicative behaviours of autistic children.' *Journal of Music Therapy 1,* 31–62.

Edwards, D. (1999) 'The role of the case study in art therapy research.' *Inscape 4,* 1, 2–9.

Frith, U. (1989) *Autism, Explaining the Enigma.* (First edition.) Oxford: Blackwell.

Howat, R. (1995) 'Elizabeth: A Case Study of an Autistic Child with Individual Music Therapy.' In T. Wigram, B. Saperston and R. West (eds) *The Art and Science of Music Therapy: A Handbook.* London: Harwood Academic.

Kanner, L. (1943) 'Autistic disturbances of affective contact.' *Nervous Child 2,* 217–250

Laverty, S. (2003) 'Hermeneutic phenomenology: a comparison of historical and methodological considerations.' *International Journal of Qualitative Methods 2,* 3, 1–29.

Levinge, A. (1990) '"The use of I and me": music therapy with an autistic child.' *British Journal of Music Therapy 4,* 2, 15–18.

McLeod, J. (2001) *Qualitative Research in Counselling and Psychotherapy.* London: Sage Publications.

Meekums, B. (1993) 'Research as an Act of Creation.' In H. Payne (ed.) *Handbook of Inquiry in the Arts Therapies: One River, Many Currents.* London: Jessica Kingsley Publishers.

National Autistic Society website. Available at www.nas.org.uk, accessed on 1 September 2009.

Oldfield, A. (1995) 'Communicating through Music: The Balance between Following and Initiating.' In T. Wigram, B. Saperston, and R. West *The Art and Science of Music Therapy: A Handbook.* (Second edition.) Amsterdam: Harwood Academic Publishers GmbH.

Oldfield, A. (2006) *Interactive Music Therapy – A Positive Approach.* London: Jessica Kingsley Publishers.

Patey-Tyler, H. (2003) 'Acknowledging Alvarez. The Use of Active Techniques in the Treatment of Children with Autistic Spectrum Disorder.' In *Community, Relationship and Spirit. Continuing the Dialogue and Debate.* (Papers from the British Society of Music Therapy (BSMT)/Association of Professional Music Therapists (APMT) Annual Conference.) BSMT Publications.

Robarts, J. (1996) 'Music Therapy and Children with Autism.' In C. Trevarthen, K. Aitken, D. Papoudi and J. Robarts *Children with Autism – Diagnosis and Interventions to Meet their Needs.* London: Jessica Kingsley Publishers.

Warwick, A. and Alvin, J. (1978) *Music Therapy for the Autistic Child.* (First edition.) Oxford: Oxford University Press.

Wigram, T. (2002) 'Indications in music therapy: evidence from assessment that can identify the expectations of music therapy as a treatment for Autistic Spectrum Disorder.' *British Journal of Music Therapy 16*, 1, 11–28.

Wing, L. (1991) 'Asperger's Syndrome and Kanner's Autism.' In U. Frith (ed.) *Autism and Asperger's Syndrome.* Cambridge: Cambridge University Press.

Woodward, A. (2003) 'Three's Company: Brief Music Therapy Intervention for an Autistic Child and her Mother.' In *Community, Relationship and Spirit. Continuing the Dialogue and Debate.* (Papers from BSMT/APMT Annual Conference.) BSMT Publications.

Woodward, A. (2004) 'Music therapy for autistic children and their families: a creative spectrum.' *British Journal of Music Therapy 18*, 1, 8–14.

Yin, R.K. (2003) *Case Study Research Design and Method.* London: Sage Publications.

Chapter 14

Unmasking Hidden Resources

Communication in Children with Severe Developmental Disabilities in Music Therapy

Cochavit Elefant

INTRODUCTION

Setting the scene

Children with severe developmental disabilities are often speechless (Iacono, Carter and Hook 1998; Siegel-Causey and Bashinski 1997); however, this doesn't mean that they have nothing to say. Unveiling the child's wishes and desires could pose special challenges for the child's caregivers, as the child may not exhibit understanding or show other communicative capabilities. Revealing the hidden communicative abilities calls for the use of different motivational and expressive means that are meaningful to the child. Music therapy can be one of the means by which communicative development can take place in children with severe developmental disabilities (Elefant 2001, 2002, 2005; Elefant and Wigram, 2005; Hill 1997; Merker, Bergstrom-Isacsson and Witt Engerstrom 2001; Wigram and Elefant 2009).

During the many years that I have worked in educational settings with children with severe developmental disabilities, children and I have engaged in musical interactions and communication, musical attunement and expressivity. This builds bonding, intimacy, and fluency in the interpersonal and intrapersonal relationship. This type of work, however, is only a part of communicative development and could easily become the only area in which the child and the therapist engage. It is important to go beyond the early interaction of the 'mother–infant' stage and develop towards other communicative areas within musical and non-musical communication, just as a child with normal development would do. In other words, the therapist can assist the child to develop independence in communication in order to voice his or her communication intentions, choice making and preferences. This may initially begin to develop within the therapy room, but later could extend beyond it.

This chapter will highlight the challenges presented by children with severe developmental disabilities when addressing the issue of communication, as in the case of children with Rett Syndrome. It will look at the results of a music therapy study intended to evaluate intentional choice making, learning abilities, non-conventional communicative behaviours and song preferences in seven young girls with Rett Syndrome (Elefant 2002).[10]

The study took place in a special education centre for children with moderate to severe special needs, aged 5–10, in a middle-class city situated in central Israel. I had worked as the music therapist in the centre for several years as part of a multidisciplinary team, engaging in individual and group music therapy, and also integrating children in the community through group music therapy.

LITERATURE REVIEW

Communication in children with developmental disabilities

Communication is a wide and complex field defined in a variety of ways, depending on reference to normal or abnormal development. As for the child with normal development, despite small differences between researchers and specialists, and some differences in definitions, there seems to be agreement on the overall stages of the development of communication. When dealing with children with developmental disabilities there are many differences between populations, pathologies and syndromes that make it unrealistic to search for any commonalties in their development of communication, and it is therefore suggested to look for alternative ways of learning and communicating (Demeter 2000; Siegel-Causey and Bashinski 1997).

10 The full text of my PhD thesis can be retrieved from www.musictherapyworld.de under 'downloads and services/dissertations'.

Traditionally, the primary focus of communicative intervention for children with developmental disabilities was to enhance speech, as well as to develop prerequisite skills believed necessary for the emergence of verbal language. However, this line of thought has now been broadened, with more emphasis on the multiple processes of communication, including expanding comprehension and finding other communicative forms of expression, such as non-conventional communicative acts (Iacono *et al.* 1998; Siegel-Causey and Bashinski 1997; Sigafoos 2000).

It is important to find the right levels of communication in a population that may not develop language skills, so as to avoid overestimation or underestimation of the child's communicative level. Overestimating the child's skills may result in communicating on a level that could lead to failure, and the reduction of his or her attempts to communicate. Underestimating the child's skills, in the case of (for example) Rett Syndrome, may result in denying the child accesses to a system of communication, thereby causing communication frustration and forcing the child either to continue relying on non-symbolic signals (Iacono *et al.* 1998) or, more often, as experience shows, to withdraw from trying to communicate.

'Potential communicative act' is a term suggested by Sigafoos *et al.* (2000), which acknowledges the possibility that existing informal and idiosyncratic behaviours could become effective forms of communication. It also acknowledges that some behaviours may be symbolic (e.g. manual sign, pointing to pictures on a communication board). In addition, the use of this term avoids the issue as to whether these actions do in fact represent 'true' (intentional) communication. It is important for the caregiver to detect and recognize when the child is communicating, and then to make sense of what the child is trying to convey (Trevarthen and Burford 1995).

The act of communication starts once the person is able to define to himself his basic wants and needs. Incorporating augmentative and alternative communication,[11] such as picture symbols and communication board, into the life of individuals with severe developmental disabilities, gives children the opportunity to communicate with their surroundings, indicating their choices and preferences. This is founded on the assumption that the capacity to make and indicate choice through some means of communication is a primary and important function for all human beings.

11 Augmentative and alternative communication (AAC) is utilized by people with limited or no speech to accommodate their communication needs. Some of the systems may include body gestures, sign language or picture symbols as augmentative communication aid.

Preferences and choices

Preference and choice as concepts and values are embodied in the principle of normalization, empowerment, quality of life and self-determination (Hughes, Pitkin and Lorden 1998). Choice making is a right, and, for most people, a cherished component of life (Bambara *et al.* 1995). It gives personal autonomy and dignity, which are essential to one's quality of life (Hughes *et al.* 1998; Nozaki and Mochizuki, 1995; Sigafoos, Laurie and Pennell 1995, 1996). The opportunity to give preference and choice are typically viewed as critical to the process of one's personal growth and fulfilment (Hughes *et al.* 1998). Unfortunately, in the lives of people with severe disabilities, preference and choice-making opportunities have been noticeably absent (Bambara *et al.* 1995). Choice making therefore relies on the development of communication to the degree that intention and need can be recognized and understood. But in order for it to succeed, the power of relationship itself should not be forgotten. Communication in general, and choice making in particular, is more than achieving a set of skills – it is a common emotional understanding between individuals (Trevarthen and Burford 1995).

Communicative abilities in individuals with Rett Syndrome

Rett Syndrome (RS) is a genetic disorder affecting mainly females (Amir *et al.* 2000). Most appear to develop normally over the first 6–18 months of life, at which point development comes to a halt, with apparent loss of acquired motor and communicative skills (Burford 2005; Einspieler, Kerr, and Prechtl (2005); Nomura, Kerr and Witt-Engerström 2005). This loss leaves the child with severe stereotypic hand movement, preventing her from participating in natural interactions, and severely restricting voluntary activity (Hagberg *et al.* 1983, Hagberg, Anuret and Wahlstrom 1993; Kerr and Witt-Engerström 2001).

As a result of the drastic regression that typically occurs in the girl with RS at Stage II of this disorder (the 'destructive stage'), there will be a change in her interactions with others and a change in their responses, expectations and expressions toward her.

When trying to locate the communicative potential of this population, a dichotomy could be found. Parents report normal pre-linguistic behaviour in their daughters until the onset of regression (Budden, Meek and Henighan 1990), while other studies argue that early development of communication is already impaired before the girls enter the first or second stage of their condition (Einspieler, *et al.* 2005; Kerr 1992). The girls lose significant communication skills, more in verbal expression than in language comprehension (Budden *et al.* 1990; Lewis and Wilson 1996); however, most of them show a strong desire to communicate by means of gaze, facial expression and body gestures.

When their condition is compared to Daniel Stern's (2000) explanation of the development of 'the five senses of self' in infancy, it seems that individuals with RS do acquire what Stern (2000) defines as ' an emergent self', 'the core self with others', 'the intersubjective self', and some may have even begun to develop 'the verbal self'. With the knowledge that a girl with RS usually experiences a largely normal development at the beginning of her life, we can presume that her primary caregiver will have interacted with her as she would with a normal baby. This means that both the child and the adult will have had the emotional experience of preverbal communication and interactions through 'affect attunement' (Stern 2000).

When a child with intellectual and developmental disability shows an ability and desire to communicate, it is important to strengthen and maintain the existing communicative interactions and to incorporate them into daily use through a formal system of communication, such as augmentative and alternative communication. Since music is greatly loved by, and is motivating for, individuals with RS (Elefant 2001, 2002, 2005; Elefant and Wigram 2005; Hadsell and Coleman 1988; Montague 1986; Wesecky 1986; Wigram 1991; Wigram and Elefant 2009), music therapy can become a valuable mediator in enhancing communication and learning in this population.

Developing communication in music therapy

A number of different models, philosophies, approaches and techniques can be utilized during music therapy. The structural form of music provides security, predictability and organization, and encourages spontaneous participation in vocalization and movement (Alvin 1976; Wigram and Cass 1996). There are therapists who predominantly use improvised music, while others use pre-composed. When following an overall client-oriented approach, the same therapist may apply both types of music, depending on the client's needs and preferences at the time of therapy.

The relationship between the therapist and the client is the basis of a successful therapeutic intervention. In the case of individuals with developmental disabilities, in particular RS, it seems that as the relationship becomes secure, they become more engaged, and extend themselves with openness and freedom (Hill 1997; Wigram 1991, 1995).

Engaging in musical communicative relationship is extremely important for individuals with RS, and within that relationship they can express some of their feelings and needs. Expressing different types of feelings enhances their motivation and the urge to learn; an important pathway to facilitate communication. Pre-composed songs can be a foundation for establishing communication in individuals with RS (Elefant 2002, 2005; Elefant and Lotan 2004; Elefant and Wigram 2005; Hetzroni, Rubin and Konkol 2002; Wigram 1991; Wigram and Cass 1996; Wigram and Elefant 2009; Wylie 1996).

Using songs with children with developmental disabilities is as natural and appropriate as a mother singing to her child.

> The songs are linguistically simple and repetitive, relying on non-verbal rather than verbal communication, reflecting the child's expressions. Dialogues are sustained when the therapist, taking the score of a composed, structured song as a base, strives, in the way she sings, to be attuned to the child's facial expression, body movement, gestures and vocalization. (Wigram and Elefant 2009 p.430)

THE STUDY

Aim

In my PhD research study, entitled 'Enhancing communication in girls with Rett syndrome through songs in music therapy', 18 familiar and non-familiar, pre-composed children's songs were presented to seven girls with RS, aged 5–10. The purpose of the study was to evaluate whether the girls had intentional choice, learning abilities and song preferences. The study also set out to gather non-verbal communication expressions (communicative acts) in an attempt to understand meaningful expressive communication (Elefant 2001, 2002, 2005; Elefant and Wigram 2005). The study took place in a special education setting for children with developmental disabilities in Israel, where at the time of the study seven girls with RS attended the school. All girls were familiar with me, from either individual or group music therapy.

The design

The research design for this study was a single-case, multiple probe design (a variant of multiple baseline design).[12] In this time-series design, each individual is viewed as a single case unit in which the comparison is within and between the individual cases (Barlow and Hersen 1984; Cooper, Heron and Heward 1987; Kazdin 1982; Kratochwill 1992). The efficacy and value of single-case design in quantitative and qualitative research has become increasingly recognized in recent years. This type of design fits well in clinical practice in education settings where the client and the researcher can work as closely as possible within a therapeutic setting. In the process involved in my study the time-frame was not predetermined, and each participant reached pre-established criteria according to her individual pace.

The procedure was such that each girl first indicated her choice of a song out of two or four picture symbols or Hebrew orthography (depending on individual ability) that represented songs about a variety of topics. The girl's choice was confirmed by randomly changing the order of the symbols, then showing them to her again and once more asking her to pick the one she wanted. The 18 songs were divided into three 'sets', with a total of six songs in each set (four familiar and two unfamiliar songs in a set). The participants showed their choice by eye gazing, or by pointing with their nose or hand. They also expressed their feelings for the music by displaying a range of communicational acts (smiling, laughing, turning head away, walking away, closing eyes, or by crying). At the stage of establishing the baseline, each girl was asked to choose a song and confirm her choice, but was told that the song would not be sung to her until later. The same procedure then took place during the intervention and maintenance period; however, this time the girls were informed that the song would be sung by the therapist (with guitar accompaniment) following the girl's confirmation. The duration of the study was eight months and included baseline, baseline probes, intervention and maintenance probes, followed by three additional maintenance trials (two, six and 12 weeks after the intervention had ended). The duration for each session was about 30 minutes and sessions were held three times per week.

12 The multiple probe design uses periodical assessment in order to evaluate learning process over time. Probes used as assessment for baseline or maintenance are measured throughout the intervention at regular intervals.

The data that emerged from two video cameras were viewed and transferred into observational sheets and analysed by means of graphs and by descriptive statistics. 'Effect size' calculations were also applied. Communicative, emotional and pathological expressions emerged through observation and analysis of the video material. These were categorized according to themes and constituted some of the qualitative aspects of this research. Qualitative findings will be only briefly referred to in this chapter.

Findings and discussion

INTENTIONAL CHOICE MAKING

The results of this study revealed that all seven participants showed lack of intentional choice making during baseline (when no songs were sung), whereas when the intervention was introduced, all participants revealed a strong ability to choose songs and to confirm their choice, demonstrating intentional choice making (Figure 14.1). The results suggest that pre-composed children's songs in music therapy have an important role in revealing such potential in a population that until recently was considered ineducable, and with pre-intentional communication. In this study the songs generated motivation that was meaningful for the child, who was then able to reveal and express her communicative capability. Further investigation is warranted to determine whether these very positive results could be generalized to the wider population with severe communication disabilities.

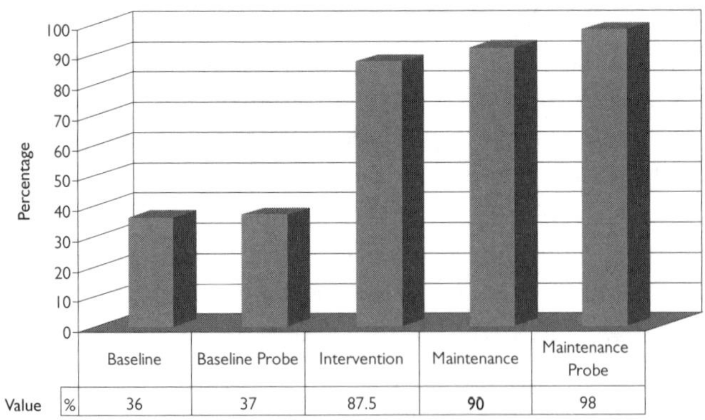

Figure 14.1: Average percentage of intentional choice making during different stages of the research

LEARNING ABILITIES

The study also revealed that all girls were able to learn, and sustained learning over time. There was an ascending trend of consistent choice making, showing that learning took place within the first few sessions during the first set of intervention. The girls were presented with six choice opportunities during each session (and were measured for intentional choice making). Figure 14.2 documents the improvement found in confirming the same song at the second viewing of the symbol cards during all sessions and with song sets. Although it is an example of findings from one girl only, it is representative of all participants in the study (Elefant 2002). The change observed ensured that learning could be considered consistent and reliable. Learning was maintained throughout intervention and during maintenance, for three months after the research had ended.

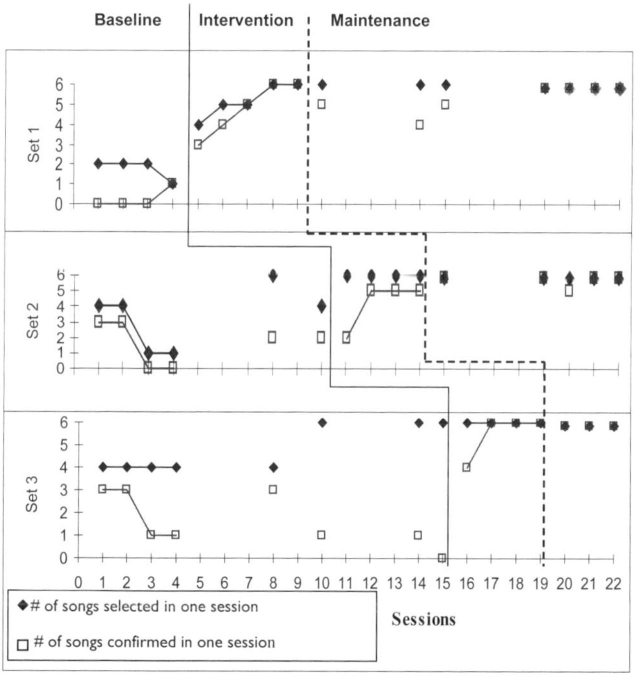

Figure 14.2: Mandy – Song selection, confirmation and learning

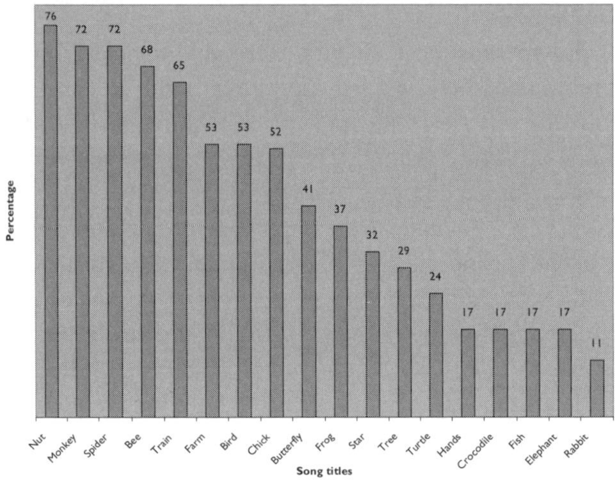

Figure 14.3: Group song preferences

SONG PREFERENCES

The research findings demonstrated that the girls as a group had distinct song preferences (Figure 14.3), and each child had clear individual likes and dislikes.

The five most preferred songs were compared to the five least preferred songs and the songs were analysed to determine what musical and non-musical features they may contain. It was not surprising to find that children with RS were able to experience preferences and could express their likes and dislikes in music, despite very severe neurological impairment, and that their preferences were consistent with the songs' musical elements.

> A general characterization of the less preferred songs would be relaxing and cradling, in the style of lullabies that are used to pacify and relax babies and young toddlers. In contrast, most of the preferred songs can be categorized as play or action songs, like those popular with children at the kindergarten level. (Wigram and Elefant 2009 432–3)

The girls' average age of seven showed that they preferred songs that are appropriate for non-disabled children of the same age group, or a little younger, but not those appropriate for a baby. This finding is important when trying to establish individual preference, and build motivation, thereby creating and enhancing meaningful experiences. This in turn empowered the participants, providing them with independence and new opportunities to strengthen themselves within their environment (Bambara *et al.* 1995; Hughes *et al.* 1998).

EMOTIONAL, COMMUNICATIVE AND PATHOLOGICAL EXPRESSIONS

An analysis of emotional, communicative and pathological expressions at a qualitative level revealed the emergence of different types of response to certain types of songs and during baseline. These responses, when examined in context, might be interpreted as understandable messages. Some expressions were frequent and exhibited by all participants, while others were unique and personal. The findings showed that it is important to identify emotional responses and different expressions that can be interpreted as communicative acts to the child by a familiar figure, such as a caregiver or a family member. Recognition of these communicative acts and understanding their intended meaning can increase shared understanding. The findings revealed the participants' 'potential communicative act' as termed by Sigafoos *et al.* (2000). The study enabled the participants to reclaim their dignity and trust as a result of regaining their lost communicative and emotional resources. 'We might say that the new-discovered skills enabled the participants to take their place in the world of humans…' (Trevarthen and Burford 1995, p.147).

It also shows that the people who are close to children with severe communication disability need to look for any communicative and emotional signs that could become meaningful to them all.

CONCLUSIONS

In this chapter I have discussed the complexity of unveiling hidden communicative resources in children with severe developmental disabilities, in particular individuals with RS. I gave an example of a research study in music therapy in which I attempted to show how communication can be studied with these children in an educational setting. I chose pre-composed children's songs because, based on my clinical experiences, I felt that when working with children with severe developmental disabilities, such pre-composed songs led to emotional and communicative expressions. The songs in the study were sung with affective attunement in synchronicity to the girls' response, in individual ways, by movements of the body and limbs, facial expressions, hand gestures and vocalizations and by the way the songs resonated with me. Each time a song was sung, it was as if a new narrative was being told, and that made it an inter-subjective experience.

By making intentional song choices and by showing their preferences, the girls became aware of their success. This type of immediate success was generalized directly into the girls' daily life. The girls began to use communication boards and devices in the classroom and at home, and within a short period their communication abilities expanded.

A research intervention in an educational setting can have many benefits to the participants involved, and it is not necessarily an isolated study in which the participants are being 'used' as subjects without gain. In the study one can see at least two important communication directions. One of them was that the girls had an opportunity to expose spontaneous communicative acts that could be utilized by everyone close to them. The other benefit was that a formal communication system, such as communication boards, was established for each girl, in which she could communicate with others and demonstrate her intentional choice making and preferences.

The multiple probe design is commonly used in naturalistic environments such as classrooms with a population of people with developmental disability (Bambara *et al.* 1995; Hetzroni, *et al.* 2002; Hetzroni and Schanin 1998; Hetzroni and Shalem 1998; Hughes *et al.* 1998; Nozaki and Mochizuki 1995; Sevcik, Romski and Adamson 1999). In this study its effectiveness and suitability for individuals with developmental disabilities and in an educational setting were re-established.

Single-case design is a suitable design for the therapist as well, as it stays close to the practice of the therapist (Aldridge 1996). The present study, a single-case design, had the flavour of therapy sessions. It took place in a natural environment, in a known setting, and in a situation familiar to the participants and the researcher. Moreover, this design was found sensitive enough to differentiate individual abilities and variables and was especially suited for evaluating whether these abilities were sustained following periods of no intervention. It is my view that the flexibility of this design makes it suitable for music therapy situations, both in research and as a practical tool to organize and measure intervention with children with developmental disabilities.

A few words are warranted about the differences between music therapy sessions in an educational centre and this type of research study which employed pre-composed songs. During music therapy sessions, song choice may be one of the activities offered, and a more flexible, client-directed approach will be employed, resulting in the use of instrumental or vocal improvisation. The music therapy sessions during the research simply took into consideration the client's 'here and now' communicative and emotional well-being and expressions. (Although there may not be any spoken language involved, I attempt to recognize any communicative or emotional signals in order to give meaning to the client's expressions.)

Some ethical issues of the research design should be considered in future studies. During baseline and baseline probes, when no songs were sung in response to the participants' choice making, the participants on occasions seemed confused, upset, bored or angry. These baseline probes may have provoked a feeling of failure, as they were being sustained concurrently with the interventions and the intervention process was disrupted repeatedly at the periodic probe measures. On the other hand, the negative effect of the baseline probes was inevitable, and this fortifies the efficacy of the intervention.

Another ethical discussion could be around the issue of the girl confirming her choice after she had already made it. This was the only way in which the study could show that the girls' choice was intentional and not by mere chance. In a 'natural' therapeutic situation, this is not recommended. Communication should not be a test. It could, however, happen that the child makes an arbitrary or unintentional choice, but this should be taken as a decision made by him or her. This in turn could help the child take control and responsibility for his or her actions.

Finally, this study suggests that with an attentive, co-operative child, good rapport between child and researcher, a familiar situation and a strong motivational factor can facilitate positive outcomes.

REFERENCES

Aldridge, D. (1996) *Music Therapy Research and Practice in Medicine.* London: Jessica Kingsley Publishers.

Amir, R.E., Van den Veyver, I.B., Schultz, R., Malicki, D.M., Tran, C.Q., Dahle, E.J., Philippi, A., Timar, L., Percy, A.K., Motil, K.J., Lichtarge, O., Smith, E.O., Glaze, D.G. and Zoghbi, H.Y (2000) 'Influence of mutation type and X chromosome inactivation on Rett syndrome phenotypes.' *Annals of Neurology.* 47, 670–679.

Alvin, J. (1976) *Music Therapy for the Handicapped Child* (Second edition.) Oxford: Oxford University Press.

Bambara, L.M., Koger, F., Katzer, T., and Devenport, T.A. (1995) 'Embedding choice in context of daily routine: an experimental case study.' *Journal of the Association for Persons with Severe Handicaps 20,* 3, 185–195.

Barlow, D.H. and Hersen, M. (1984) *Single Case Experimental Designs.* Concord, MA: Simon & Schuster.

Budden, S., Meek, M. and Henighan, C. (1990) 'Communication and oral-motor function in Rett syndrome.' *Developmental Medicine and Child Neurology 32,* 51–55.

Burford, B. (2005). 'Perturbations in the development of infants with Rett disorder and the implications for early diagnosis.' *Brain and Development 27,* Suppl. 1, S3–S7.

Cooper, J.O., Heron, T.E and Heward, W.L. (1987) *Applied Behavior Analysis.* Columbus, OH: Merrill.

Demeter, K. (2000) 'Assessing the developmental level in Rett syndrome: an alternative approach?' *European Child and Adolescent Psychiatry 9,* 227–233.

Einspieler, C., Kerr, A. M. and Prechtl, H. F. (2005). 'Abnormal general movements in girls with Rett disorder: the first four months of life.' *Brain and Development 27*: Suppl. 1, S8–S13.

Elefant, C. (2001) 'Speechless yet Communicative: Revealing the Person behind the Disability of Rett Syndrome through Clinical Research on Songs in Music Therapy.' In D. Aldridge, G. Di Franco, E. Ruud and T. Wigram (eds) *Music Therapy in Europe.* Rome: ISMEZ.

Elefant, C. (2002) 'Enhancing communication in girls with Rett syndrome through songs in music therapy.' Unpublished PhD thesis. Aalborg University, Denmark.

Elefant, C. (2005) 'The Use of Single Case Designs in Testing a Specific Hypothesis.' In D. Aldridge (ed.) *Case Study Designs in Music Therapy.* London: Jessica Kingsley Publishers, 145–162.

Elefant, C. and Lotan, M. (2004) 'Rett Syndrome: dual intervention – music and physical therapy.' *Nordic Journal of Music Therapy 13,* 2, 172–182.

Elefant, C. and Wigram, T. (2005). 'Learning ability in children with Rett syndrome.' *Brain and Development 27,* 97–101.

Hadsell, N.A. and Coleman, K.A. (1988) 'Rett syndrome: a challenge for music therapists.' *Music Therapy Perspectives 5,* 52–56.

Hagberg, B., Aicardi, J., Dias, K. and Ramos, O. (1983) 'A progressive syndrome of autism, dementia, ataxia, and loss of purposeful hand use in girls. Rett's syndrome: Report of 35 cases.' *Annals of Neurology 14,* 471–479.

Hagberg, B., Anuret, M. and Wahlstrom, J. (eds) (1993) *Rett Syndrome – Clinical and Biological Aspects.* ('Clinics in Developmental Medicine' No. 127.) London and Cambridge: MacKeith Press/Cambridge University Press.

Hetzroni, O., Rubin, C. and Konkol, O. (2002) 'The use of assistive technology for symbol identification by children with Rett syndrome.' *Journal of Intellectual and Developmental Disability 27,* 1, 57–71.

Hetzroni, O. and Schanin, M. (1998) 'Computer as a tool in developing emerging literacy in children with developmental disabilities.' (Hebrew journal). *Issues in Special Education and Rehabilitation Journal 13,* 1, 15–21.

Hetzroni, O. and Shalem, O. (1998) 'Augmentative and alternative communication – the use of picture symbols in children with autism.' (Hebrew journal). *Issues in Special Education and Rehabilitation Journal 13,* 1, 33–43SS.

Hill, S.A. (1997) 'The relevance and value of music therapy for children with Rett syndrome.' *British Journal of Special Education 24,* 3, 124–128.

Hughes, C., Pitkin, S.E. and Lorden, S.W. (1998) 'Assessing preferences and choice of persons with severe and profound mental retardation.' *Education and Training in Mental Retardation and Developmental Disabilities 33,* 4, 299–316.

Iacono, T., Carter, M. and Hook, J. (1998) 'Identification of intentional communication in students with severe and multiple disabilities.' *AAC Augmentative and Alternative Communication 14,* 102–114.

Kazdin, A.E. (1982) *Single-case Research Design.* Oxford: Oxford University Press.

Kerr, A.M. (1992) *Communication in Rett Syndrome.* London: Rett Syndrome Association UK.

Kerr, A.M. and Witt-Engerström, I. (2001) 'The Clinical Background to the Rett Disorder.' In A.M. Kerr and I. Witt-Engerström (eds) *Rett Disorder and the Developing Brain.* Oxford: Oxford University Press.

Kratochwill, T.R. (1992) *Single-case Research Design and Analysis.* Hillsdale, NJ: Lawrence Erlbaum Associates.

Lewis, J.E. and Wilson, C.D. (1996) *Pathways to Learning in Rett Syndrome.* Telford, Shropshire: Wozencroft Printers.

Merker, B., Bergstrom-Isacsson, M. and Witt Engerstrom, I. (2001) 'Music and the Rett disorder: the Swedish Rett Center survey.' *Nordic Journal of Music Therapy 10,* 1, 42–53.

Montague, J. (1986) *Music Therapy in the Treatment of Rett Syndrome.* Glasgow: National Rett Syndrome Association.

Nomura, Y., Kerr, A. and Witt-Engerström, I. (eds) (2005) 'Rett syndrome: early behaviour and possibilities for intervention.' *Brain and Development 27,* Suppl. 1, S101.

Nozaki, K. and Mochizuki, A. (1995) 'Assessing choice making for persons with profound disabilities: a preliminary analysis.' *Journal of the Association for Persons with Severe Handicaps 20,* 3, 196–201.

Sevcik, R.A., Romski, M.A. and Adamson, L.B. (1999) 'Measuring AAC interventions for individuals with severe developmental disabilities.' *AAC Augmentative and Alternative Communication,* 15, 38–44.

Siegel-Causey, E. and Bashinski, S.M. (1997) 'Enhancing initial communication and responsiveness of learners with multiple disabilities: a tri-focus framework for partners.' *Focus on Autism and Other Developmental Disabilities 12,* 2, 105–120.

Sigafoos, J. (2000). 'Communication development and aberrant behavior in children with developmental disabilities.' *Education and Training in Mental Retardation and Developmental Disabilities 35,* 2, 168–176.

Sigafoos, J., Laurie, S. and Pennell, D. (1995) 'Preliminary assessment of choice making among children with Rett syndrome.' *Journal of the Association for Persons with Severe Handicaps 20,* 175–184.

Sigafoos, J., Laurie, S. and Pennell, D. (1996) 'Teaching children with Rett syndrome to request preferred objects using aided communication: two preliminary studies.' *Augmentative and Alternative Communication 12,* 88–96.

Sigafoos, J., Woddyatt, G., Tucker, M., Robers-Pennell, D. and Pittendreigh, N. (2000) 'Assessment of potential communication acts in three individuals with Rett Syndrome'. *Journal of Development and Physical Disabilities, 12,* (3), 203–216.

Stern, D.N. (2000) *The Interpersonal World of the Infant.* (Revised edition.) New York: Basic Books.

Trevarthen, C. and Burford, B. (1995) 'The central role of parents: how they can give power to a motor impaired child's acting, experiencing and sharing.' *European Journal of Special Needs Education 10,* 2, 138–148.

Wesecky, A. (1986) 'Music therapy for children with Rett Syndrome.' *American Journal of Medical Genetics 24,* 253–257.

Wigram, T. (1991) 'Music Therapy for a Girl with Rett's Syndrome: Balancing Structure and Freedom.' In K. Bruscia (ed.) *Case Studies in Music Therapy.* Gilson, NH: Barcelona Publishers.

Wigram, T. (1995) 'A Model of Assessment and Differential Diagnosis of Handicap in Children through the Medium of Music Therapy.' In T. Wigram, B. Saperston and R. West (eds) *The Art and Science of Music Therapy: A Handbook.* Chur, Switzerland: Harwood Academic Publishers GmbH.

Wigram, T. and Elefant, C. (2009). 'Therapeutic Dialogues in Music: Nurturing Musicality of Communication in Children with Autistic Spectrum Disorder and Rett Syndrome.' In S. Malloch and C. Trevarthen (eds) *Communicative Musicality: Exploring the Basis of Human Companionship*. Oxford: Oxford University Press, 423–445.

Wigram, T. and Cass, H. (1996) 'Music therapy within the assessment process for a therapy clinic for people with Rett syndrome.' Paper presented at the Rett Syndrome World Conference in Sweden.

Wylie, M.E. (1996) 'A case study to promote hand use in children with Rett syndrome.' *Music Therapy Perspectives 14*, 83–86.

Chapter 15

Facing the Challenge

A Music Therapy Investigation in the Evidence-based Framework

Katrina McFerran and Jennifer Stephenson

INTRODUCTION

Setting the scene

This chapter will describe a music therapy study conducted in partnership by two academics from Australian universities. Katrina McFerran is a qualitative researcher in music therapy and Jennifer Stephenson favours quantitative research in special education. This collaboration was established in response to media interest in challenges to the efficacy of music therapy in the Australian context, framed as a controversial practice (Stephenson 2004). Music therapy is well represented in the Australian special schools, with a recent survey finding that 41 per cent of Victorian special schools employ music therapists (Booth 2004). The opportunity to explore the role of music therapy in special education from an evidence-based perspective was of interest to both the authors and to professionals in both disciplines.

Evidence-based practice (EBP) was introduced originally to medical settings, but has spread throughout the healthcare and education fields. Broadly speaking, EBP places an emphasis on the use of evidence from sound research studies, along with clinical expertise and the perspectives of the individual receiving treatment in the processes for making decisions about clinical practice (Schlosser and Raghavendra 2004). This set of beliefs is grounded in a desire to support best practice and to distinguish interventions supported by 'evidence' from 'popular' practice, that is, interventions that are widely supported by schools but not founded on empirical research. Music therapists have acknowledged the dominance of the evidence-based approach in both medical settings (Edwards 2002) and special education (McFerran and Stephenson 2007), although some authors have challenged the values underpinning any approach that privileges one form of knowing over all others both in music therapy (Aldridge 2003; Edwards 2005) and in education literature (Lincoln 2005).

Special education in Australia has an easy relationship with EBP because, unlike mainstream education, it is primarily derived from the scientific tradition of applied behaviour analysis. The field has always placed a strong emphasis on the use of practices for which there is empirical evidence of the type valued in the EBP model. There are literally hundreds of empirical studies demonstrating the efficacy of a wide range of special education practices (Alberto and Troutman 2006; Westling and Fox 2003). Although there is an emerging interest in qualitative work to examine more closely the dynamics of particular situations, only a small body of literature has been published (Brantlinger, *et al.* 2005). Within the field of music therapy, some researchers have advocated applied behaviour analysis as a preferred research methodology (Hanser 2005; Standley 1996). However, the discipline also has a rich tradition of case study, descriptive and qualitative work.

LITERATURE REVIEW

There is a wealth of music therapy literature that music therapists perceive as valid evidence supporting the use of music therapy in educational settings (Daveson and Edwards 1998). Wigram (1993) identified 453 articles in the music therapy literature that focused on special education, and Jellison (2000) identified 148 papers on music research in the field of childhood disabilities. In addition, a review by Gold, Voracek and Wigram (2004) identified two empirical studies related to students with intellectual disability. Although hundreds of articles have addressed music therapy in special education, it is apparent that the vast majority of studies and reviews do not fulfil the criteria of rigorous empirical design required by EBP (Odom *et al.* 2005; Schlosser, Wendt and Sigafoos 2007).

If music therapy services are to be included in educational programmes for students with severe disabilities, it is not unreasonable for educators to look for evidence that music therapy can contribute to the achievement of educational objectives. Special educators acknowledge that music therapists are specifically trained to design individualized music treatment plans for children with severe disabilities (Ockelford 2000) and recognize the potential of music therapy to provide a motivating context for communicative interaction (Stephenson 2006). Both Ockleford (2000) and Bunt (2003) have argued that music therapy and music education may overlap in the middle ground between music education goals and therapeutic goals. Although music therapy is reportedly focused on the well-being of students with severe disabilities (Meadows 2002), in practice it often addresses issues to do with the overall development of the child, and educational goals are frequently incorporated into the individualised learning programme goals addressed in music therapy programmes implemented in schools.

For many students with severe disabilities, objectives in individual music therapy programmes are likely to focus on communication and social interaction skills (Westling and Fox 2003). Music therapy literature demonstrates a consistent focus on the development of intentional and presymbolic communication for these students (Stephenson 2006). Perry's (2003) qualitative investigation described the effect of different levels of intentional and pre-intentional communication on musical interactions in therapy and emphasized the importance of turn-taking and joint attention in music therapy interaction. Recent empirical studies include Elefant and Wigram's (2005) report on improved communication skills in girls with Rett Syndrome, and Kim, Wigram and Gold's (2008) study of increased levels of joint attention in children with autism. Specific observable behaviours that provide evidence of the proposed educational outcomes resulting from music therapy have not yet been detailed sufficiently in the music therapy literature.

THE STUDY

Aim

In response to the debate about the benefits of music therapy for children with severe disabilities in school settings, and the consensus between music therapists and special educators about the high priority of developing communication skills for students with severe disabilities, the authors agreed to conduct an investigation together. The hypothesis was that students with severe disabilities would produce more communicative acts during music therapy interventions than when they were interacting with the same therapist during other activities without music or singing. The independent variable in this study was the presence or absence of music. The dependent variables were the communicative behaviours of the participants in the two contrasting conditions. The study was intended explicitly to explore the use of music during interaction, given that music is an essential component of music therapy.

Participants

Four students and four music therapists participated in the study. A detailed analysis of results from one student will be presented in this chapter to illustrate the challenges faced in using the evidence-based framework to investigate individual music therapy. The student was a nine-year-old boy with severe intellectual disability, cortical visual impairment, spastic quadriplegia and cerebral palsy, as well as other health impairments. He used a wheelchair for mobility and had limited movement of his arms, but was able to activate a switch with his elbow if it was suitably positioned.

The music therapist had worked with the participant for two years prior to the study and had an established relationship. Her music therapy approach is representative of humanistic styles of working with this population commonly practised in Australia. The therapy was provided in individual 20–30 minute sessions on a weekly basis, with the music therapist participating regularly in team meetings that worked towards the development of individualized learning plans.

Research design

Within the EBP approach, carefully designed single subject designs can provide trustworthy evidence, particularly when designs are replicated with participants with different characteristics and by different research groups (Odom *et al.* 2005). Single subject research has a strong focus on the individual, and so provides a means of measuring the effects of a specific set of conditions on individuals, as opposed to measuring mean effects on a large group.

The study utilized an ABAB design to explore what effect the use of music by the music therapist had on the communication interactions between adult and child. At a simple level it could be argued that if music does not make a difference to the communicative behaviour of a student, the benefit of adding music as an element within the music therapist–student interaction could be questioned for that student. The collection of detailed data on student and therapist behaviour allows us to examine in certain detail the interaction between student and therapist and how the use of music might change the interaction.

In this study, the A phase comprised sessions where the therapist interacted with the student around favourite activities (such as a vibrating mat triggered by a switch and the reading of favourite books), other than those related to music and the use of the voice for singing. The B phase comprised sessions where the therapist interacted using music therapy methods grounded in familiar songs and improvised duets, including the student's use of a switch to produce musical sounds. In both contexts, the therapist encouraged communicative responses and the student's engagement in the activities.

Measures

We collected video recordings of five non-music sessions, followed by five music sessions, and then, because of the student's illness, only three further non-music sessions followed by three music sessions. Each video recording was coded to extract data relating to form of communication used, turn-taking, and the apparent function of each turn. The coders judged the degree of intent of actions by the student. A very conservative definition of intentional communication was used in order to ensure good inter-rater reliability, relying on clear evidence of the student alternating their eye gaze between the therapist and an action or activity, with at least two gaze shifts (e.g. look at object, make eye contact with therapist, look at object again).

These elements and their operational definitions were drawn from the literature on the communicative behaviour of persons with severe disabilities and their communication partners. We used the work of Brady *et al.* (1995), McLean *et al.* (1991), and Ogletree, Wetherby and Westling (1992) for classification of and operational definitions for the forms, functions and communicative intentionality of participants. The coding of the behaviour of the music therapist drew on the work of Carter (2003), Nind, Kellett and Hopkins (2001), and Sigafoos *et al.* (1994) for likely antecedents of child communicative behaviour and the opportunities that communication partners may offer, as well as the range of responses that the partner might make in response to child behaviour. The music therapy interventions drew heavily on improvizatory frameworks, and the music therapist's actions were coded using common terminology such as 'mirroring' and 'matching' (Wigram 2004), as well as imitating (Bruscia 1987).[13]

In order to establish that the coding and thus the data collected were reliable, we used two coders. These coders were initially trained on video not associated with the project, and coding was further refined by discussion and recoding of some of the video taken in the project. Both coders were provided with a manual that supplied guidelines for coding and definitions of each code, and they worked independently of one another. To establish inter-coder reliability, 25 per cent of each of the non-music sessions and 25 per cent of five of the eight music sessions were coded by both of the coders.

Findings and discussion

RELIABILITY

The first consideration from an EBP perspective is that the data coded were shown to be reliable. Typically in single-subject designs coding for the presence or absence of events, 80 per cent agreement[14] is considered acceptable. In a study such as this with large amounts of complex data, lower levels of reliability are acceptable (Kennedy 2005). For this study we have used 75 per cent as an acceptable level of reliability, and the reliability of some aspects of coding was poor.

Data on the music therapist were generally reliable, and she was coded as consistently offering opportunities for the student to maintain attention to the therapist and the activities she was presenting. This was achieved through a range of behaviour – touching the student, speech, making sounds, and making music. Other strategies occurred less frequently, perhaps related to the slow pace of work with this boy, with each session comprising only three or four different activities. The data on the student were much less reliable, and coders could not agree on either form or intent (see Table 15.1). Most of the disagreements related to the coding of facial expression, which was probably affected by the student's cortical vision impairment.

13 The authors are happy to share the data collection tool upon request.

14 Calculated by using the formula: agreements divided by agreements, plus disagreements, multiplied by 100.

Table 15.1: Reliability summary

	Mean reliability (%)	Range
RMT form	85.2	70.8 to 93.2
Student form	70.19	34.4 to 97
RMT turns	79.1	71.1 to 90.9
Student turns	80.2	72 to 100
Student intent	69.1	47.3 to 100
Student function	84.7	45.5 to 100
RMT opportunities provided	90.2	80 to 97.7
RMT responses to student	82.9	50 to 100

Although the student's behaviour could not generally be coded reliably, there was agreement that very few student behaviours were intentionally communicative according to our conservative definition. The poor reliability of data on this student's actions is itself evidence of the ambiguity of his behaviour (Nicholas, Geers and Rollins 1999).

Analysis of results

As is usual for single-subject designs, the results were graphed and inspected visually for indications of effects (Kennedy 2005). To demonstrate a clear clinical effect for the use of music, the data points in the two conditions (interaction with and without music) should show no, or minimal, overlap. Since the data on opportunities for communicative responses offered by the music therapist were reliable, and there was reliable coding for goal-directed responses from the student for 10 of the 15 sessions where reliability data were available, we present this data (see Figure 15.1) as an example of the overall results. Similar patterns of overlapping data points were obtained when we graphed the number of music therapist's turns against student's turns and music therapist's opportunities provided against all responses. The data on the forms of switch activation and vocalizing were also reasonably reliable. (Switch data were reliable for all except one session and vocalizations for all except two sessions.) We present those data as well (see Figure 15.2).

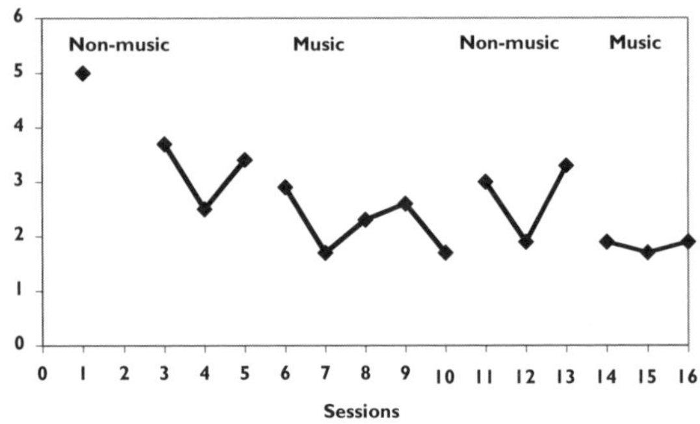

Figure 15.1: Opportunities provided per one goal-directed behaviour

Notes:

- There is no data point for Session 2 (no music) because the student slept through most of this session.
- Data for goal-directed behaviour are unreliable for sessions 1,11 and 12 (non-music) and Sessions 7 and 9 (music).

The student's engagement increased after the first two non-music sessions and he used more switching and vocalizations to interact with the therapist around favourite books and sensory toys. During initial non-music sessions it is possible that the child was confused by the presence of the music therapist without music – an interpretation that is supported by his behaviour. The re-introduction of music then resulted in some highly interactive sessions; however, these achievements were moderated by some less responsive sessions in the music condition that were equivalent to the most interactive of the non-music sessions. This scenario was repeated in the second set, and the overlap between conditions makes evidence for the impact of the musical elements unconvincing.

It can be argued that there is a small advantage for music sessions in that the student was more responsive to opportunities offered in the music sessions (although only marginally so). The lowest rate of vocalizations occurred in non-music sessions, and the highest rates in music sessions. Similarly, the higher rates of switch activations were also in music sessions. These results should all be treated with due caution because of the low reliability of some of the data.

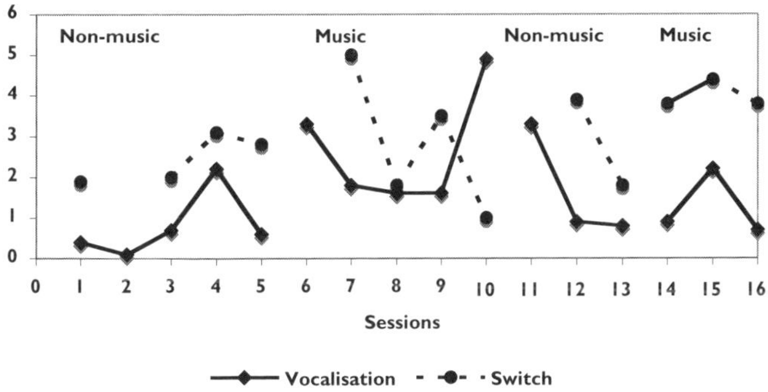

Figure 15.2: Vocalizations and turns with switch activations per minute

Notes:

- The switch was not available in Session 2 (no music), Session 6 (music) and Session 11 (no music).
- Some switch events were multiple activations in close proximity that our coders could not separate as separate events.

These data could be seen as reflecting the importance of the interaction between the student and the therapist, and could suggest that for this boy the type of activity around which the interaction occurred was less important than the interaction itself. In both music and non-music sessions the therapist worked to engage his attention, whether with switch toys or with musical activities. Similarly, in both sessions she offered some opportunities for greeting or farewelling, choosing, requesting and responding to questions. The difficulty of interpreting the student's behaviour (exemplified by the difficulties in reliable coding) must also present difficulties to the therapist working with him and attempting to be appropriately responsive to his behaviour.

Limitations

There are several limitations to this study. The coding of the data was not always reliable. Issues with inter-rater reliability in future studies might be addressed with the use of consensus coding instead of independent coding, as this strategy is commonly used in special education studies investigating students with more severe disabilities (Carter 2003).

In future studies with students functioning at this level of emerging intentional communication, it may be helpful to gain some insight into particular forms that regular communication partners regard as communicative. The Inventory of Potentially Communicative Acts (Sigafoos *et al.* 2000) is a tool designed to gather this kind of information, which would allow more detailed coding of idiosyncratic student behaviour that partners may respond to.

The use of a control condition that reflects the intervention in every way except the musical interaction is a strain for music therapy investigations, and potentially other creative arts interventions, and in this study there was no attempt to prescribe the music therapist's behaviour closely except for the use of music. The therapeutic relationship is integral to the expected benefits from interventions, and the separation of the music alone is more similar to music psychology studies than the investigation of music therapy. This study does endorse, however, that enjoyable and relaxed interaction sequences that are non-directive and engaging may be a motivating context for interaction, even without the music (Nind and Hewett 1988).

The profound nature of the student's disability resulted in an inconsistent state of being, and his capacity appeared to vary due to internal physical states. In further work it may be helpful to code behaviour state (a measure of the degree of alertness of the student) as one of the dependent variables, as has been done in exploring the communication behaviour of children with severe disabilities in other contexts (Arthur 2004).

CONCLUSION

Although the analysis of the data from this dyad failed to demonstrate a clear clinical effect for the use of music, it has allowed us to identify some of the problems associated with this methodological approach and has demonstrated that it is possible to code reliable data reflecting music therapist and student interaction. This information is particularly valuable with the increasing interest in video microanalysis emerging in the field of music therapy (Wosch and Wigram 2007). Further work with more refined coding schemes and more individualized analysis of student behaviour appears to be a promising direction for empirical investigation of the impact of music therapy on this population.

REFERENCES

Alberto, P.A. and Troutman, A.C. (2006) *Applied Behaviour Analysis for Teachers.* (Seventh edition.) Upper Saddle River, NJ: Paul H. Brookes.

Aldridge, D. (2003) 'Staying close to practice: which evidence, for whom, by whom.' [Electronic version.] *Music Therapy Today 4.* Available at www.musictherapyworld.de, accessed on 18 December 2007

Arthur, M. (2004) 'Patterns amongst behaviour states, socio-communicative and activity variables in educational programmes for students with profound and multiple disabilities.' *Journal of Developmental and Physical Disabilities 16,* 125–149.

Booth, R. (2004) 'Current practice and understanding of music therapy in Victorian special schools.' *Australian Journal of Music Therapy 15,* 64–75.

Brady, N.C., McLean, J.E., McLean, L.K. and Johnston, S. (1995) 'Initiation and repair of intentional communication by adults with severe to profound cognitive disabilities.' *Journal of Speech and Hearing Research 38,* 1334–1348.

Brantlinger, E., Jimenez, R., Klingner, J., Pugach, M. and Richardson, V. (2005) 'Qualitative studies in special education.' *Exceptional Children 71,* 195–207.

Bruscia, K. (1987) *Improvisational Models of Music Therapy.* Philadelphia, PA: Charles C. Thomas.

Bunt, L. (2003) 'Music therapy with children: a complementary service to music education?' *British Journal of Music Education 20,* 179–195.

Carter, M. (2003) 'Communicative spontaneity in children with high support needs who use augmentative or alternative communication systems. II: Antecedents and effectiveness of communication.' *Augmentative and Alternative Communication 19,* 155–169.

Daveson, B. and Edwards, J. (1998) 'A role for music therapy in special education.' *International Journal of Disability, Development and Education 45,* 4, 449–455.

Edwards, J. (2002) 'Using the evidence-based medicine framework to support music therapy posts in healthcare settings.' *British Journal of Music Therapy 16,* 1, 29–34.

Edwards, J. (2005) 'Possibilities and problems for evidence-based practice in music therapy.' *The Arts in Psychotherapy 32,* 4, 293–301.

Elefant, C. and Wigram, T. (2005) 'Learning ability in children with Rett syndrome.' *Brain and Development 27,* Suppl. 1, 97–101.

Gold, C., Voracek, M. and Wigram, T. (2004) 'Effects of music therapy for children and adolescents with psychopathology: a meta-analysis.' *Journal of Child Psychology and Psychiatry 45,* 1054–1063.

Hanser, S.B. (2005) 'Applied Behaviour Analysis.' In B. Wheeler (ed.) *Music Therapy Research.* (Second edition.), Phoenixville, PA: Barcelona Publishers, 306–318.

Jellison, J. (2000) 'A Content Analysis of Music Research with Disabled Children and Youth (1975–1999): Applications in Special Education.' In *Effectiveness of music therapy procedures. Documentation of research and clinical practice* (Third edition.) Silver Spring, MD: American Music Therapy Association, 199–264.

Kennedy, C.H. (2005) *Single-case Designs for Educational Research.* Boston, MA: Allyn & Bacon.

Kim, J., Wigram, T. and Gold, C. (2008) 'The effects of improvisational music therapy on joint attention behaviours in autistic children: a randomized control study.' *Journal of Autism and Developmental Disorders 38,* 9, 1758–1766.

Lincoln, Y.S. (2005) 'Institutional Review Boards and Methodological Conservatism: The Challenges to and from Phenomenological Paradigms.' In N.K. Denzin and Y.S. Lincoln (eds) *The SAGE Handbook of Qualitative Research.* (Third edition.) London: SAGE.

McFerran, K. and Stephenson, J. (2007) 'Music therapy in special education: do we need more evidence?' *British Journal of Music Therapy 20,* 2, 121–128.

McLean, J.E., McLean, L.K.S., Brady, N.C. and Etter, R. (1991) 'Communication profiles of two types of gesture using nonverbal persons with severe to profound mental retardation.' *Journal of Speech and Hearing Research 34*, 294–308.

Meadows, A. (2002) 'Approaches to music and movement for children with severe and profound multiple disabilities.' *The Australian Journal of Music Therapy 13*, 17–27.

Nicholas, J., Geers, A.E. and Rollins, P.R. (1999) 'Inter-rater reliability as a reflection of the ambiguity in the communication of deaf and normally-hearing children.' *Journal of Communication Disorders 32*, 121–134.

Nind, M. and Hewett, D. (1988) 'Interaction as curriculum.' *British Journal of Special Education 15*, 2, 55–57.

Nind, M., Kellett, M. and Hopkins, V. (2001) 'Teachers' talk styles: communicating with learners with severe and complex learning difficulties.' *Child Language Teaching and Therapy 17*, 143–159.

Ockelford, A. (2000) 'Music in the education of children with severe or profound learning difficulties: issues in current UK provision, a new conceptual framework, and proposals for research.' *Psychology of Music 28*, 1197–1217.

Odom, S., Brantlinger, E., Gersten, R., Horner, R.H., Thompson, B. and Harris, K. (2005) 'Research in special education: scientific methods and evidence-based practices.' *Exceptional Children 71*, 137–148.

Ogletree, B.T., Wetherby, A.M. and Westling, D.L. (1991) 'Profile of the prelinguistic intentional communicative behaviours of children with profound mental retardation.' *American Journal on Mental Retardation 97*, 186–196.

Perry, M. (2003) 'Relating improvisational music therapy with severely and multiply disabled children to communication development.' *Journal of Music Therapy 40*, 3, 227–246.

Schlosser, R.W. and Raghavendra, P. (2004) 'Evidence-based practice in augmentative and alternative communication.' *Augmentative and Alternative Communication 20*, 1–21.

Schlosser, R.W., Wendt, O. and Sigafoos, J. (2007) 'Not all systematic reviews are created equal: considerations for appraisal.' *Evidence-based Communication Assessment and Intervention 1*, 138–150.

Sigafoos, J., Roberts, D., Kerr, M., Couzens, D. and Baglioni, A.J. (1994) 'Opportunities for communication in classrooms serving children with developmental disabilities.' *Journal of Autism and Developmental Disorders 24*, 259–279.

Sigafoos, J., Woodyatt, G., Keen, D., Tait, K., Tucker, M., Roberts-Pennell, D. and Pittendreigh, N. (2000) 'Identifying potential communicative acts in children with developmental and physical disabilities.' *Communication Disorders Quarterly 21*, 77–86.

Standley, J.M. (1996) 'A meta-analysis on the effects of music as reinforcement for educational/therapy objectives.' *Journal of Research in Music Education 44*, 2, 105–133.

Stephenson, J. (2004) 'Controversial practices in the education of students with high support needs.' *Journal of Research in Special Education Needs 4*, 1, 58–64.

Stephenson, J. (2006) 'Music therapy and the education of students with severe disabilities.' *Education and Training in Developmental Disabilities 41*, 290–299.

Westling, D.L. and Fox, L. (2003) *Teaching Students with Severe Disabilities.* (Third edition.) Upper Saddle River, NJ: Merrill Prentice Hall.

Wigram, T. (1993) 'Music Therapy Research to Meet the Demands of Health and Educational Services.' In M. Heal and T. Wigram (eds) *Music Therapy in Health and Education.* London: Jessica Kingsley Publishers.

Wigram, T. (2004) *Improvisation: Methods and Techniques for Music Therapy Clinicians, Educators and Students.* London: Jessica Kingsley Publishers.

Wosch, T. and Wigram, T. (eds) (2007) *Microanalysis in Music Therapy: Methods, Techniques and Applications for Clinicians, Researchers, Educators and Students.* London: Jessica Kingsley Publishers.

Summary and Conclusions

Vicky Karkou

The examples of research and practice included in this book do not exhaust the many ways in which arts therapists can work with children and young people in school environments. They do, however, indicate key areas of practice and overall trends. Some of the main themes emerging from the chapters of this book relate to:

- the needs of the clients
- the type of work
- theoretical influences
- research evidence
- collaboration.

CLIENT NEEDS

The children that arts therapists are involved with in mainstream schools face difficulties that range in severity from risk of developing mental health problems (but not regarded as requiring specialized input and support) to more serious difficulties – for example, loss and/or trauma as a result of natural disasters (e.g. tsunami), abuse or neglect.

The contributors to this book have described therapeutic interventions with children who are facing bullying, violence or disaffection. These contributors in particular are arts therapists practising in the USA and the UK – see the work of Suzi Tortora in Chapter 1, Lynn Koshland in Chapter 2 and Toby Quibell in Chapter 6. It is possible that this reflects broader social issues faced by children and young people in these countries. It is also possible that particular therapeutic interventions are tied up with government policies and associated funding that aim to tackle these issues.

In some cases, arts therapies are seen as a stable and supportive intervention for children in transition. They can be offered as a way of enabling children to move from primary to secondary schools, or from centres and specialized services for excluded children back to mainstream education (see Chapter 4), or as a way of managing the constant changes caused by children's turbulent family lives (see Chapter 9).

Several contributors understand the needs of the children and young people they work with from an educational perspective, and describe their clients as having 'additional support needs' or 'specific learning difficulties'. Successful therapy interventions with this client group are perceived as those that have an impact in terms of improved learning outcomes (see, for example, Chapters 7 and 8).

When arts therapists are placed in special schools, they often work with children with varied and multiple needs. Particularly important seems to be the contribution of arts therapies in working with children with autism: four case studies that refer to this client group have been included in the book (Chapters 10–13). Rett Syndrome, cerebral palsy and severe (pervasive) developmental difficulties also seem to be relevant client groups, as indicated by three of the research studies presented (Chapters 11, 14 and 15). In all cases, the key theme that emerges within special education seems to be the contribution made by arts therapies in supporting effective communication and relationship building.

TYPE OF WORK

Contributors to the book have described therapeutic interventions lasting from six sessions to three years. The majority of the interventions are short-term, maybe because of limited funding, the school ethos and the need to follow the school calendar. Sessions can take place in a number of different locations:

- mainstream or special classroom
- special facilities inside the school, e.g. the school gym, dance or drama studios, the music room, etc.
- services outside the school, e.g. private practice, pupil referral units, etc.

The book covers a number of different interventions according to the severity and type of need of the children involved, as well as the overall therapeutic aim. Alongside typical therapy work involving children over a period of time, there are projects that target whole schools through theme-based interventions (see, for example, Chapter 6). There are also projects that aim towards mental health promotion through educational programmes for teaching staff and direct therapeutic work for young people at risk (see, for example, Chapter 3). This latter type of work encourages practitioners to shift their attention from dealing with children's mental health problems to engaging with early intervention and prevention of mental illness. In most chapters of this book, the duration of this type of therapy tends to be fairly short (up to 12 sessions), reflecting the needs of the children involved. At times it may also reflect small-size project work, time-limited funding and/or session work.

Supportive therapy is also proposed as a viable option that is sometimes more appropriate than in-depth therapy; Chapter 9 of this book has presented arguments in favour of supportive therapy as a stable and non-challenging intervention for a looked-after child in transition to a long-term foster home. Other cases in which supportive work may be preferred can involve children in acute distress, children recovering from physical illness, children faced with stressful environmental factors (e.g. having to deal with a court case or having to return to an abusive family situation). In these cases, work can focus primarily on arts making, and the therapist can offer him- or herself as a consistent and benign presence, but without attempting to offer interpretations, explore deep traumas, etc.

THEORETICAL INFLUENCES

The arts therapists contributing to this book conceptualize their work in a number of different ways. In order to do this, they often draw upon specific theories that have emerged from their own discipline. For example, amongst the dance movement psychotherapists there are regular references to Marian Chace and her interactive model. Dramatherapists talk about embodiment, projection and role, a model developed by Sue Jennings, one of the pioneers of dramatherapy in the UK. Others acknowledge the value of mirroring and affective attunement as a non- or preverbal empathetic response to the child with learning difficulties that fosters therapeutic communication. Interestingly enough, arts therapists go beyond their own disciplines and make additional references to theoretical underpinning from psychotherapeutic literature, including:

- person-centred therapy (Rogers)
- psychodynamically informed practices (Freud, Klein, Erikson, Winnicott and Bowlby; also Alvarez)
- group theory (Foulkes, Yalom)
- solution-focused therapy (Selekman)
- developmental psychology (Stern and Trevarthen).

As discussed in the introduction to the book, there were historical links between the child-led principles prevalent in schools in Britain up until the 1990s and the emergence of arts therapies. These links probably explain why some arts therapists prefer to draw upon principles from *Rogerian person-centred therapy.* With memories of child-led education still in existence amongst teaching staff, arts therapists can relatively easily translate their work back to educational practice, using ideas and principles that are understood and at times shared by their teaching colleagues.

Psychodynamically-informed practices remain relevant to arts therapies in schools, particularly when children with more severe psychological needs are concerned. For example, there are stronger references to psychodynamic thinking when arts therapists work with looked-after children or children facing trauma or loss, or in work challenging adolescent defences. Within a mainstream context, arts therapists may refer to Freud, Klein, Erikson, and often ideas from Winnicott, while in special education the work of Alvarez seems of particular value. Attachment theory (Bowlby in particular) appears to be the most frequently referenced theoretical influence amongst arts therapists. Its popularity may be due to its clear and well researched foundation, the overt links that it makes between internal experience, behaviour and environment, and its wide use within a number of different professions. Like principles borrowed from person-centred therapy, attachment theory offers guidance for arts therapies sessions. It also provides a language in which arts therapists can discuss with other colleagues (e.g. social workers, educational psychologists, speech and language therapists) joint strategies on how best to support their young clients.

As group work is fairly common within the school environment, *group theory* can be another asset in the arts therapist's toolkit. Considering group dynamics that are relevant not only to arts therapies group session but also to the school environment as a whole can offer insights into the school ethos, and consequently better enable arts therapists to contextualize a child's experience.

Given the short duration of most of the interventions included in this book, particular theoretical frameworks that might support brief work are not sufficiently explored. With the exception of the dramatherapist Genevieve Smyth and her efforts to integrate *solution-focused therapy* (Selekman) with brief dramatherapy (Chapter 5), no contributor has really engaged with this topic. It is clear that there is a need for further work in the area.

Within a special education context, arts therapists repetitively refer to *developmental psychology*, and to Stern and Trevarthen in particular. The contribution of Stern and Trevarthen is particularly relevant to arts therapists because they attach significance to intersubjective experiences that rely on physical, musical and visual interactions and the associated emotionality of these interactions. Non- and pre-verbal communication with emotional content lies at the heart of arts therapy work with children with learning disabilities and severe learning disabilities in particular.

However one of the most important theoretical contributions of this book is in a clear call to develop therapeutic models that are directly linked with school practice. Suggestions are made to include creative synergies between arts therapies theory and practice and educational principles and concepts. It is possible that this call, filtered through experience and articulated through extensive research work, reflects a genuine need to develop solid and context-appropriate therapeutic frameworks. Consequently, the models already suggested, i.e. educational music therapy (Chapter 7) and art educational therapy (Chapter 8), deserve further attention and development in order to strengthen the theoretical foundations of the work undertaken by arts therapists in schools.

RESEARCH EVIDENCE

Next to theoretical contributions, this book also makes a case for the need for research. As discussed in the introduction and demonstrated in all the chapters following, there are multiple ways in which arts therapists can engage with research activities. Types of studies included in this book draw upon:

- qualitative methodologies with a case study design
- arts-based research
- quantitative methodologies with randomized controlled trials and experimental designs
- mixed methodologies and designs.

Qualitative methodologies are quite common, especially when arts therapists are interested in evaluating the process of the work through case study designs. Useful qualitative methodologies include grounded theory and hermeneutic phenomenology. The most common research methods used include interviews, participant observations and questionnaires, alongside collections of images, music, video recordings, stories or other dramatic enactments. Studies that follow case-study designs remain very close to practice, as a number of the contributions to this book show (see, for example, Chapters 1, 4, 11 and 13). Furthermore, the roles of the practitioner and the researcher become one. The new amalgamated role of the practitioner/researcher (most contributors of this book fall into this category) has certain characteristics. The practitioner/researcher is:

- curious about human nature
- keen to go into more depth in working with young clients
- respectful of the views of the child, parents, teachers, other professionals and key workers
- committed to improving his or her practice
- ready to let go of practices that do not seem to work.

In these terms, routine evaluation becomes an integral part of practice. Furthermore, qualitative studies can contribute towards the generation of theory and practice-based evidence that can be directly fed back to the field through published work. For arts therapists starting with a new client group, it is vital to look at the type of work already completed by colleagues, the main difficulties encountered and the key themes emerging, besides consulting studies that argue about effectiveness. Critical appraisal skills are important here in order to make decisions on the quality of these publications, their relevance to practice and their value for a particular client and/or client group.

Closely connected with qualitative methodologies is *arts-based research*. In this book, arts therapists are reminded that research does not have to be removed from the creative components of the work. Frances Prokofiev in Chapter 9 offers a good example of focusing on images created by one of her clients as a central point of her research work. Immersing and dialoguing with the artwork that has been created within the sessions or in response to the sessions can offer valuable information about the development of the therapeutic work. Bringing the arts at the centre of the therapist's attention with an appropriate conceptual frame a valuable research activity directly linked with therapeutic work.

Finally, a number of the contributions to the book have strong quantitative components, either in *mixed methods designs* or in *pure quantitative studies*. Two randomized controlled trials are included, that look at the effectiveness of dance movement psychotherapy and dramatherapy for children and adolescents (see Chapters 3 and 6, respectively). In both cases, arts therapies were seen as effective in reducing anxiety and depression. Two research studies with experimental designs are included, that look at particular aspects of music therapy, e.g. the role of pre-composed songs for children with Rett Syndrome (Chapter 14) and the value of music in therapeutic interaction with children with severe learning difficulties (Chapter 15).

The contribution of *quantitative studies* lies largely in the fact that 'hard' evidence is generated. Hard evidence is often required to achieve professional recognition and to further support the professional role of arts therapists in schools. However, quantitative studies can also offer interesting insights in the therapeutic work. In Chapter 14, for example, Elefant's study on the value of using pre-composed songs with clients with Rett Syndrome can have direct implications on music therapy practice. Similarly, in Chapter 15, McFerran and Stephenson's study raises interesting points relating to whether it is the therapeutic relationship or the presence of music that is mainly responsible for therapeutic change.

In all cases, the ability to source and critically appraise available research studies is a key aspect of contemporary therapy and relevant to arts therapists working in schools. The need to generate further evidence is also essential, either through routine evaluations of practice or through engaging with larger research studies. Often the latter cannot be done without sufficient training, experience, time and money. Collaboration with other professionals who may possess complementary skills is therefore strongly recommended, as the following section shows.

COLLABORATION

Collaboration is the final key theme emerging from this book. It relates to collaboration between individual arts therapists and:

- arts therapies teams
- arts therapies tutors/supervisors/researchers and trainees
- teachers, head teachers and teaching staff
- educational psychologists, counsellors, psychiatrists, social workers and health professionals.

Collaborations that 'work' have the potential to contribute towards cultural shifts that question the tradition of the sole practitioner who works on his or her own in the back room, the basement or the kitchen area, forgotten and disconnected from the rest of the school. Collaboration can enable arts therapists to bypass the fact that they are usually the only arts therapist employed in a particular setting, and create real or virtual links with other professionals. In the UK there are active 'arts therapies in education' groups that can provide such network opportunities. In this book (Chapter 3), Karkou, Fullarton and Scarth offer an example of a successful collaboration that involved arts therapists from different disciplines (e.g. dance movement psychotherapists and art therapists) coming together to work on the one project in different roles (e.g. therapist, researcher, teacher, manager) and consequently making different contributions. Collaborations between qualified arts therapists and trainees can also be of value, as demonstrated in Lynn Koshland's contribution to the book in Chapter 2.

Links with teachers and teaching staff supporting children in schools are even more important, as they can facilitate therapeutic work. The special educational needs co-ordinators (SENCO) in England, or guidance tutors in Scotland, are of key importance for arts therapists, as they can send referrals and help monitor and jointly support children in distress; so too are other professionals involved in the care of children and young people, such as educational psychologists, counsellors, psychiatrists and health professionals.

Collaboration can also take the shape of creating partnerships between arts therapies and other services. These can include partnerships with:

- services and local authority
- existing mental health services available in schools

- artists and other creative agents
- independent research teams, or research teams situated within university institutions.

Further work is needed to integrate arts therapies within learning support units, pupil referral centres, Children and Adolescent Mental Health Services and organizations operating within schools that offer psychological support for children in need, such as The Place2Be,[15] Kids' Company,[16] etc.

Effort is also required regarding the development of posts and career structures within the school system as a whole. Although often financial reasons and existing power dynamics determine the extent to which arts therapists can be employed within the educational system, arts therapists can help shift the balance and engage more actively with the educational system. This can be supported by being clear about the psychological needs of children who can benefit from arts therapies, and the type of interventions the therapist can offer. Articulated theoretical frameworks and practices that are evidence-based and appropriately evaluated are also important. Finally, we have suggested that it is possibly time for arts therapists to develop ways of working that are tailored around the school culture. This can create better chances of offering integrated services that will promote the role of arts therapists in schools, and ultimately benefit children and young people in need.

15 The Place2Be is a charity that supports children's emotional well-being in primary schools in the UK (see www.theplace2be.org.uk).

16 Kids' Company is also a charitable organization with a similar remit to The Place2Be, offering therapeutic support to vulnerable children in and out of the school environment (see www.kidsco.org.uk).

The Contributors

Jo Christensen MA (Dramatherapy) DipDth, PGCE, BA (Drama and Theatre Studies)
Jo began using drama in education, prisons, children's homes, and with a variety of community groups. For ten years she worked in secondary education, teaching drama and also establishing and delivering dramatherapy in Emotional and Behavioural Units. Jo now works across Cornwall as a freelance dramatherapist and writer. Most recently she has been involved in project work in Nepal. She aims to continue to research and apply the use of metaphor as a tool for transformation and education.

Cochavit Elefant PhD (Music Therapy), M Mus, B Mus, BA (Music Therapy)
Cochavit is Associate Professor of Music Therapy at the Grieg Academy, University of Bergen, Norway. She has worked for many years in special schools in Israel and USA as a music therapist and is currently researching people with Parkinson's disease in Music Therapy. Her recent research in community music therapy will appear in an upcoming book, *Where Music Helps: Community Music Therapy in Action and Reflection,* co-authored by her with by G. Ansdell, B. Stige and M. Pavlicevic (in press).

Ailsa Fullarton MPhil, PG Dip (Art Therapy), PG Cert, BA (Hons)
Ailsa has over ten years' experience of working with children and young people with autism spectrum disorder (ASD). Since she qualified as an art therapist in 2003 she has worked in both specialist and mainstream educational settings across Scotland. Ailsa has been highly active in the field of the arts therapies in Scotland and has been the chair of the Scottish Arts Therapies Forum (SATF).

Vicky Karkou PhD, M Ed, PgDip (Dance Movement Therapy), B Ed Sc (Hons)
Vicky is a senior lecturer and the programme leader for the MSc in Dance Movement Psychotherapy at Queen Margaret University, Edinburgh. She has worked in mainstream and special schools as an arts therapist and a teacher, and has researched and published in the area. Her first book (co-authored with P. Sanderson) is entitled: *Arts Therapies: A Research-Based Map of the Field* (Elsevier 2006).

Lynn Koshland MA (Dance Therapy), ADTR, MSW (Movement Studies), LCSW, MALS, BS (Early Childhood Ed)
Lynn works as a dance movement therapist and licensed clinical social worker in elementary school and senior centres. She is a recipient of a research grant from the Marian Chace Foundation of the American Dance Therapy Association and numerous other grants. She is published in *American Dance Therapy Journal*, in a book *Music Therapy with Hospitalized Children. A Creative Arts Child Life Approach*, and in her *PEACE* programme booklet. Lynn recently returned from teaching her programme in Seoul, Korea, 2008 for the Korean Dance Therapy Association.

Katrina McFerran PhD, RMT (Registered Music Therapist), B Mus (hons)
Katrina McFerran is a senior lecturer and music therapy researcher at the University of Melbourne in Australia. Her clinical and research interests focus on young people with physical, intellectual and mental health difficulties, and particularly on the use of music to facilitate personal development. She

has published and presented internationally for the past decade, and has now published on this topic with *Adolescents, Music and Music Therapy: Methods and Techniques for Clinicians Educators and Students.* (Jessica Kingsley Publishers, forthcoming).

Unnur G. Ottarsdottir PhD, MA (Art Therapy), ATR (Registered Art Therapist), B Ed (Teacher Education)
Unnur practises art educational therapy (AET) and art therapy in her private practice and conducts research at the Reykjavik Academy. She holds a PhD in art therapy from the University of Hertfordshire, an MA in art therapy from the Pratt Institute in New York and a B Ed degree in teaching from the Iceland University of Education. Since 1990, Unnur has practised art therapy in several organizations, including schools in Iceland where she has also worked as a teacher, a special educational teacher and an art educational therapist. Currently, she is the chair of the Icelandic Art Therapists' Association.

Emma Pethybridge PG Dip (Music Therapy, Nordoff-Robbins), BA (Joint Hons)
Emma has worked for NHS Lothian in the Children's Music Therapy Service since graduating with a Postgraduate Diploma in Music Therapy (Nordoff-Robbins) from the University of Edinburgh in 2004. In 2005 she received funding from the Youth Music Initiative (Scottish Arts Council) through the Department of Community Services in East Lothian to extend the service and to develop time-limited group work projects in schools in East Lothian.

Frances Prokofiev MA (Art Psychotherapy), Dip AT, BA (Fine Art)
Frances developed her practice as an art therapist in a London primary school and currently teaches on the MA in Art Psychotherapy Research for the Northern Programme for Art Psychotherapy based in Sheffield. She is also a visiting lecturer at Goldsmiths' College, University of London. She is engaged in doctoral research at Goldsmiths', focusing on the role of the art process in art therapy with children. She has also written on art therapy in schools and children's groups.

Toby Quibell PhD, Dip Psy, Dip (Dramatherapy), PGCE
Toby is director of The Learning Challenge and a visiting fellow at the University of Newcastle. The Learning Challenge is based in the Northeast of England, working to develop and deliver critical, creative and therapeutic curriculum offers in school, especially where social inequalities have had a corrosive effect on personal aspiration. Toby's research interests are group work, school ethos and enquiry-based approaches to learning.

James Robertson, MPhil, PGCE, Dip Music Therapy (Nordoff-Robbins), Dip Mus Ed
James is the Programme Leader of the MSc Music Therapy (Nordoff-Robbins) at Queen Margaret University, Edinburgh. He has worked in both music therapy and music education; his main research interest has focused on the similarities and differences between these two fields, and this has led to the concept of educational music therapy. His clinical practice is now situated in forensic mental health.

Susan Scarth MCAT (Dance Movement Therapy), SrDMP, CMA
Susan has 20 years' experience as a dance movement psychotherapist, lecturer, trainer (in the UK and abroad) and supervisor, combined with a proactive profile in the professional body ADMP UK. She is currently a lecturer at Queen Margaret University, Edinburgh on the MSc Dance Movement Psychotherapy Programme, with special interest in abuse and trauma, parent/child health and adult mental health.

Genevieve Smyth MA, PgDip (Dramatherapy) BA (Drama and English)
Genevieve works in child and adolescent community mental health in NHS Borders. As a dramatherapist for 18 years, she has established new UK services and offered training in Eastern

Europe, the US, Canada and Asia; as well as running a private practice, she is chair of Dramatherapy Scotland, a guest lecturer with Queen Margaret University and the Scottish link person for the British Association of Dramatherapists. Genevieve is published in Phil Jones' *Drama as Therapy*, published by Routledge.

Jennifer Stephenson PhD, Postgrad Dip (Special Education) Dip SKTC, Dip Ed, B Sc
Jennifer is an Associate Professor in Special Education at the Macquarie University Special Education Centre at Macquarie University (Sydney, Australia). Her research interests are the education of students with severe disabilities, particularly in the area of communication development and in the use of controversial and unproven practices in special education settings.

Fuyuko Takeda MA (Art Therapy), PG Dip, BA
Fuyuko is an art therapist and a member of the Art Therapy in School Service. She has been working in a variety of educational settings in Southeast England, specializing in children and young people with autistic spectrum disorders. She is currently working in mainstream and special schools in London.

Jo Tomlinson MA (Music Therapy), LGSM, PGCE, GMus
Jo has worked in special needs and mainstream schools in Cambridgeshire since 1995, employed by Cambridgeshire Music. Jo lectured on the music therapy course at Anglia Ruskin University from 2001 to 2002 and was Head Music Therapist for Cambridgeshire Music from 2002 to 2005. She has presented papers at numerous music therapy conferences.

Lynn Tytherleigh MA (Dramatherapy), B Ed (Hons)
Lynn works as a dramatherapist with children and young people in a wide variety of schools in Bedfordshire. Lynn has considerable experience of working with individuals and groups with learning disabilities, including autism. She also teaches drama and is a personal tutor for students in a school for children with additional needs, where she promotes student self-advocacy, therapeutic and person-centred approaches, and support for parents.

Suzi Tortora Ed D, MA (Dance Therapy), BC-DTR, CMA, LCAT
Suzi is a licensed dance movement psychotherapist and a certified Laban nonverbal communication analyst. She has a private practice, works extensively with children with Autism Spectrum Disorders, and has created dance therapy programs for medically ill children in hospital settings. Suzi lectures and provides training programs about her *Ways of Seeing* program nationally and internationally. She has published papers about her therapeutic and nonverbal communication analysis work with children, parent-infant dyads, and Autism Spectrum Disorders. Suzi's book, *The Dancing Dialogue: Using the Communicative Power of Movement with Young Children*, was published in 2006 by Paul H. Brookes Publishing Co.

Hilda Wengrower PhD, DMT
Director of the Masters at Barcelona University in Spain and a lecturer at the Hebrew University in Jerusalem, Hilda co-edited with Sharon Chaiklin *La Vida es Danza. El Arte y la Ciencia de la Danza Movimiento Terapia* (Gedisa, 2008) and *The Art and Science of Dance Movement Therapy. Life is Dance* (Routledge, 2009). Within her rich clinical experience, her areas of special interest and research are: intergroup conflict, artistic inquiry, creativity, clinical and non-clinical applications of DMT. She has published articles and chapters and is guest editor of the *Journal Babel* of the Universidad Bolivariana de Chile.

Subject Index

Achenbach System of Empirically Based Assessment (ASEBA) 66, 120
Action GroupSkills Intervention (AGI) 19, 115–26
effectiveness 124–6
programmes and activities 121–2
structure of sessions 121–2, 123
adolescent development 61–3
'affect attunement' 208, 212–13
American Music Therapy Association 130
Angel Child, Dragon Child (Surat) 50
Argentina, dance movement therapy 45
art educational therapy (AET) 19, 156–7
art psychotherapy 9
see also art therapy; arts therapies in school
art therapy
concept terminology 9
extent of use in schools 12–13
integrating into school curriculum 146–9
literature reviews 218–20
in specific learning difficulties sessions within mainstream schools 145–58
working with children with autistic spectrum disorders 199–200, 217–29
see also arts therapies in schools
arts education, cf. arts therapies 10–11
arts therapies in schools
background and history 10–12
collaboration between professions 278–9
contributions towards mental health promotion programmes 63–4
importance of settings 11–13
needs of clients 271–2
recognition and professionalization 10, 11–13
theoretical influences 273–5
types of work 272–3
use of short-term interventions 17, 94–5
arts-based research 277
attachment theory 62, 76
Australia and arts therapies, use of music therapy 21–2
autism spectrum disorder (ASD) and arts therapies 20–1, 179–81, 197–8, 231–2
existing interventions 198–200
psychotherapeutic treatments 180
relationship building activities 20
use of art therapy 199–200, 217–29
use of dance movement therapy 179–93
use of dramatherapy 201–14
use of music therapy 231–40
awareness of others, use of dance movement therapy 49, 55–6

behaviour changes
data analysis methods 51–5, 70–9
transformative stages 101, 106, 110–11
Bloomberg School of Public Health (John Hopkins University) 179–80
body awareness techniques 32
Body—Mind Centering (Cohen) 32
breath awareness techniques 32, 37
breathing exercises in group work 185
brief therapy *see* solution-focused brief therapy
British Art Therapy Association (BAAT), alliance with NUT 13
building relationships *see* relationship building activities
bullying in schools
extent of problem 43–4
from perspective of perpetrator 17, 33–6, 39–40
literature reviews 29, 44–5
use of dance movement psychotherapy 27–40
use of dance movement therapy 45–57
use of prevention programmes 45–57
'Bullyproof Your School' programme 45

Center for Autism and Developmental Disabilities Epidemiology 180
Chace Approach (dance movement therapies) 67–9, 184, 273
change analysis *see* behaviour changes
chasing games 208–9
child and adolescent development 61–3
choice making 250, 255
client needs 271–2
Cochrane Collaboration 15
collaboration between professions 278–9
Colombo's Children's Book Society 97–8
communication in children with severe developmental difficulties 244–7
use of music therapy 247–55
control groups 80
criminality pathways 44
cueing 208
Current Approaches to Drama Therapy (Lewis and Read Johnson) 101

dance movement psychotherapy
background and literature 28–9
concept terminology 9
evaluation methods 17–18, 65–6, 67–9, 71–9
history of use in schools 12
in mental health promotion programmes 17–18, 59–81
structure of sessions 37
'Ways of Seeing' programme 29–32, 32–40
see also arts therapies in schools; dance movement therapy

dance movement therapy
  concept terminology 9
  evaluation studies 186–93
  in mainstream schools 17, 45–57
  in special schools 179–93
  see also arts therapies in schools
The Dancing Dialogue (Tortora) 34–5
developmental psychology 274, 275
disaffection in schools 115–16
dramatherapy
  background and literature reviews 86–7
  concept terminology 9
  as contribution to 'emotional curriculum' 18–19, 114–26
  with people with autistic spectrum disorders 201–14
  processes and transformative stages 101, 106, 110–11
  use for relationship building 197–214
  use of solution-focused brief therapy 18, 97–112
  within learning support units 18, 85–95
  see also arts therapies in schools
Dramatic Approaches to Brief Therapy (Gersie) 98
dreams 219–20

East Lothian Council (Scotland), Educational Music Therapy initiatives 134–43
Educational Music Therapy 19, 129–43
  background and literature review 130–2
  definitions 131
  development of new models 131–3
  evaluation studies 134–43
Embodiment, Projection and Role (EPR) 20, 87, 273
emotional regulation
  through dance movement therapy 49, 55–6
  through dance music psychotherapy 32
'empathic reflection' 181, 185–6, 193
evidence-based practice
  concerns about evaluation methodologies 14–16
  frameworks for music therapy 259–68
exclusion practices, role of student support units (SSUs) 85–6

fantasy and daydreaming 219–20
'five-story self structure model' (Casson) 89, 93–4

foster care, school–based arts therapies for children in transition 161–74
Freudian theories 62
Friedman test 73

game playing 199
Gatehouse Study 117
group development patterns 62–3, 76
group theory 274–5
group work 71–81, 116, 210–11, 213
  Action GroupSkills Intervention (AGI) 19, 115–26

habit formation 207
Health Professions Council (HPC) 10
  on dance movement psychotherapy 12
hierarchy of evidence 15
'holding' techniques 192–3

Iceland and arts therapies 146–58
'identity crisis' 62–3
imagination and autism 219–20
  evaluating art therapy interventions 220–9
  sensory aspects 228
imitation techniques 20, 185–6
  literature reviews 181–3
intensive solution focused therapies *see* solution-focused brief therapy
intentional choice making 250, 255
Inventory of Potentially Communicative Acts (Sigafoos) 268

kinaesthetic empathy 20, 36–7, 185–6, 191

Labian Movement Analysis (LMA) 30, 69, 181
Labyrinth project 64, 65–81
  aims and objectives 65
  design 65–6
  intervention methods 66–9
  participants 69–70
  study findings and discussion 70–4
learning support units, and dramatherapy 18, 85–95
Lög um grunnskóla 146
looked-after children
  literature reviews 161–2
  school-based arts therapies 161–74

mainstream schools 17–20, 27–174
  art therapy interventions 145–58
  dramatherapy interventions 18, 97–112, 114–26
  ethos and culture 116–18
  interventions for specific learning difficulties 145–58
  learning support units 18, 85–95
  levels of disaffection 115–16
  mental health promotion programmes 17–18, 59–81
  new collaborative models of working 19, 131–3, 133–43
  preventing pupil exclusions 18, 85–95
  support for looked-after children 19–20, 161–74
  use of Action GroupSkills Intervention (AGI) 19, 115–26
  use of an educational music therapy initiatives 131–43
  using short-term interventions 18, 94–5, 97–112
  working with bullying and violence 17, 27–40, 43–57
Marian Chace Foundation 46, 57
mask use 92, 107
mental health promotion programmes 17–18, 59–81
  background and literature review 60–4
  contribution of arts therapies 63–4
mirroring techniques 20, 181, 189–91
  in dance movement therapy 183–5, 185–6
  outcomes 192
mixed methods research 277
modelling techniques 45
'moratorium' (Erikson) 62
Movement Signature Impressions (MSI) 32–3
music education 130
music therapy 12
  evidence-based practice (EBP) frameworks 259–68
  new models of work 19, 131–3
  societal frameworks 130
  training for teachers 140
  use for children with autism 231–40
  use for children with severe developmental difficulties 243–55, 259–68
  see also educational music therapy

National Autistic Society 217, 232
National Literacy Trust 85
National Qualifications online 60
National Union of Teachers (NUT) 13
needs of client groups 271–2
'Nonreader's Hassle Log' (Goldstein) 50–2

object use 207
observational tools
'Nonreader's Hassle Log' (Goldstein) 50–2
Ways of Seeing daily note forms 32–3
one-to-one relationship building 208
The Owl and the Woodpecker (Wildsmith) 49

partnership working 278–9
PEACE school violence prevention programme 45–57
peer relationships
in adolescence 61–3
bullying and violence 29, 43–5
person-centred therapy (Rogers) 274
Personal and Social Education (PSE) 60
personal, social and health education (PSHE) 60
play therapy 199
'potential communicative act' (Sigafoos) 245, 268
pre-composed songs 21, 248, 253–4
Pretend Play Test 221–7
problem-solving skills development, through use of dance movement therapy 49–50, 55–6
professionalization of art therapies 10–11, 12
and collaborative working practices 278–9
projective techniques, and relationship building 207, 213
PSHE *see* personal, social and health education (PSHE)
puppet use 91–2, 107

Qualifications and Curriculum Authority 60
qualitative methodologies 276
quantitative studies 277
'Quit It' programmes 45

randomized controlled trials (RCTs) evaluations 15, 116, 277
of Action GroupSkills Intervention (AGI) 116, 120126
of dance movement psychotherapy 17–18, 65–6, 67–9, 71–9
reciprocal cueing 208
recording tools, 'Nonreader's Hassle Log' (Goldstein) 50
relationship building activities
use of dance movement therapy 49–50, 55–6
use of dramatherapy 200–14
working within special schools 20, 197–214
research on arts therapies practice in schools 14–16, 275–7
concerns about evaluation methodologies 14–16
use of control groups 80
Rett syndrome 20–1, 244, 246–7
role engagement 210, 213

school settings 11–13
impact on arts therapies practice 13–14
research on arts therapies practice 14–16
see also mainstream schools; special schools
Scotland
additional support for learning initiatives 129–30
use of an educational music therapy initiatives 131–43
self-control skills, and dance movement therapy 48, 55–6
self-disclosures 122
severe developmental disabilities
communication through music therapy 243–55, 260–1, 260–8
'shared relationships' 209
short-term interventions 17, 94–5, 97–112
'six-part story-making model' (Lahad) 87
socialization 44–5
solution-focused brief therapy 18, 24, 97–112, 274
literature review 98–101
'special educational music therapy' (Goll) 130
special schools 179–268
art therapy work 199–200, 217–29
dance movement therapies 20, 179–93
music therapies 20–1, 231–40
for children with severe developmental difficulties 243–55
symbolic and imagination work 20–1, 210, 213, 219–29
Sri Lanka and dramatherapy interventions 18, 97–112
SSUs *see* student support units (SSUs)
sterotypical habits 207
'stop–go' games 210–11
STOP-GAP Methods 101
storytelling methods 87
student support units (SSUs), and dramatherapy 18, 85–95
supportive therapy 273
symbolic work 20–1, 210, 213

T-tests on behaviour changes 52–3
TEACCH approach 204, 217, 232, 234
team working *see* collaboration between professions
theoretical influences, overview 273–5
transformative stages of changing behaviours 101, 106, 110–11
'transitional objects' 76
types of work 272–3

violence in schools 17, 43–5
use of dance movement therapy 45–57
use of prevention programmes 45–57

'Ways of Seeing' programme 29–32
evaluation studies 32–40
Wilcoxon test 73

Youth Music Initiative (Scottish Arts Council) 132–43
evaluation and findings 141–2

Author Index

Achenbach, T. 66, 120, 150, 157
Adamson, L. 254
Adler, J. 180
Ainsworth, M.D.S. 32, 62
Aitken, K. 180, 183
Al Ruaie, T. 187
Alberto, P.A. 260
Aldridge, D. 254, 260
Aldridge, F. 146, 162
Alvarez, A. 180, 192, 199, 211, 214
Alvin, J. 64, 199, 207, 232, 235–6, 247
American Music Therapy Association 130
Amir, R.E. 246
Andsell, G. 204, 233
Anuret, M. 246
Anzalone, M. 32
Appleton, V. 146–7
Arthur, M. 268
Asperger, H. 231

Baines, E. 117
Baker, M.J. 210
Bambara, L.M. 246, 254–5
Barkley, R.A. 150, 157
Barlow, D.H. 249
Baron-Cohen, S. 219, 221, 232
Bartenieff, I. 32
Bashinski, S. 243–5
Batmanghelidjh, C. 115
Beardall, N. 29, 45
Beaumont, M. 149–50
Bell, J. 103
Bell, R.M. 117
Bergman, S. 29
Bergstrom-Isacsson, M. 243
Bernstein, P. 28, 30–1
Bettelheim, B. 218, 231
Biklen, S.K. 33
Bion, W.R. 192–3
Bishop, D. 220
Blatchford, P.B. 117
Blau, B. 184
Blos, P. 62, 64, 68
Blotzer, M.A. 198
Bogdan, R. 33
Bolton, G. 121
Bolton, P. 232
Bond, L. 117–18
Booth, R. 259
Botvin, G.J. 117
Bowlby, J. 62, 64, 68, 76, 86, 161
Boxall, Majorie 86
Brady, N.C. 263
Braken, B.A. 120
Brantlinger, E. 260
Brigg, G. 205
Bromfield, R. 199
Brown, S. 199, 209, 232
Bruscia, K.E. 130–1, 264
Budden, S. 246–7
Bunt, L. 11, 232, 261
Burford, B. 245–6, 246, 253
Bush, J. 16, 149
Butler, H. 118

Carrette, J. 201
Carter, M. 243, 245, 263, 267
Case, C. 162, 172
Casson, J.W. 87, 89
Castelli, F. 218
Cattanach, A. 98
Cesaroni, L. 198, 206
Chaiklin, H. 31, 184
Chaiklin, S. 67–9, 181, 184, 192
Chesner, A. 201, 204–5, 210, 214
Chester, K.K. 130–1
Chilcote, R. 146
Christie, D. 117
Clarkson, P. 197, 208
Coe, R. 14
Cohen, B.B. 32
Cohen, D. 238
Coleman, K.A. 130, 247
Cooper, J. 249
Corbin, J. 150
Costello, A. 220
Coyeman, M. 45
Craig, F. 219
Crenshaw, D.A. 27
Crimmens, P. 16, 201–2, 205
Crowly, R.J. 86

Dalley, T. 149
Daniel, S. 183
Darrow, A. 130
Daveson, B. 260
Davies, P. 14
Dawson, G. 182
Demeter, K. 244
Dent-Brown, K. 94
DfE 85
DfES 117
Diamond, N. 180
Diamond, S. 101
DiCenso, A. 116
DoH 59
Dover-Councell, J. 151
Dubowski, J. 16, 65, 208–9, 218, 220
Durlak, J.A. 61, 67

Edgerton, C. 232
Edwards, J. 260
Einspieler, C. 246–7
Elefant, C. 21, 243–4, 247–8, 261
Elkin, F. 44
Ellickson, P.I. 117
Elliot, R. 203, 205
Elton, R. 115
Emunah, R. 64, 68, 72, 76, 101, 121
Erfer, T. 180
Erickson, F. 33
Erikson, E. 62, 64, 68, 72
Evans, K. 16, 63, 72, 76, 199, 208–9, 218–19

Faggiano, F. 116
Farnan, L.A. 130
Fehlner, J.D. 149
Field, T. 192
Fischman, D. 45
Flay, B. 117
Fonagy, P. 15
Fontana, D. 11
Fox, L. 260–1
Foxcroft, D.R. 116

Freud, S. 62
Fried, P. 43–5, 53
Fried, S. 43–5, 53
Frith, U. 231
Fuchs, T. 64

Galpert, L. 182
Garber, M. 198, 206
Gascho-White, W. 130
Geddes, H. 148
Geers, A.E. 265
Gersie, A. 64, 68, 72, 98
Gilbert, A.G. 28, 31
Gilroy, A. 15, 164–5
Glasman, J. 10–11, 64, 70
Glick, B. 46, 50–1, 53–4, 56–7
Glover, S. 118
Glovinsky, I. 32
Godfrey, C. 118
Gold, C. 64, 68, 214, 260–1
Goldstein, A.P. 44, 46, 50–1, 53–4, 56–7
Goleman, D. 44
Goll, H.H. 130, 140
Goodall, P. 149
Gottfredson, D.C. 117
Gould, J. 218
Grabner, T.E. 53
Grainger, R. 202, 204
Greenspan, S.I. 32, 180, 198–202, 210
Griggs-Drane, E.R. 130
Groenlund, E. 64, 68, 72
Grossman, G.S. 149

Hadsell, N.A. 247
Hagberg, B. 246
Hallam, S. 117
Halprin, D. 28
Hanney, L. 146, 147
Hanser, S.B. 260
Hargreaves, D. 14
Harvey, S. 149
Hautala, P. 149
Heal, M. 15
Heathcote, D. 121
Heine, C.C. 130
Hendricks, S. 199
Henighan, C. 246–7
Henley, D. 149
Heron, T. 249
Hersen, M. 249
Hervey, L. 45, 53
Hesse, E. 32
Hetzroni, O. 248, 254
Heward, W. 249
Hewett, D. 263, 268
Hill, S. 243, 248
Hillman, J. 218
Hobson, R. 198
Hodges, S. 199
Holland, J. 60, 70, 70–1

Hook, J. 243, 245
Hopkins, V. 263
Hoskyns, S. 232
Howat, R. 232
Hoxter, S. 162
Hughes, C. 246
Hybal, L. 117

Iacona, T. 243, 245
ICD-10 179

Janert, S. 199, 208–9
Janesick, V. 33
Jellison, J. 260
Jennings, S. 10, 20, 64, 68, 72, 87, 89, 92, 99, 121, 200–1, 204–8, 210–12
Jensen, P. 61
Jeong, Y.J. 64, 68, 72
Johnson, D.R. 45, 146–7
Johnston, T.C. 60
Jones, P. 65, 100–1, 104, 108–9, 111, 201
Jonsson, C. 183
Jordan, R. 201
Josefi, O. 199

Kalish, B. 180, 183–5, 192, 199
Kalmanowitz, D. 146, 172
Kanner, L. 218, 231
Karkou, V. 10–14, 63–5, 70, 81, 217, 220
Kazdin, A.E. 249
Kellett, M. 263
Kemmelmeyer, K.J. 130
Kennedy, C.H. 264–5
Kern Koegel, L. 210
Kerr, A.M. 246–7
Kim, J. 261
Knill, P.J. 228
Koch, S. 64, 68, 72, 77
Koegel, R.L. 210
Kolvin, I. 116, 124–5
Konkol, O. 248
Kornblum, R. 29, 45, 53
Koshland, L. 29, 44, 46–53, 55–6
Kozlowska, K. 146, 147
Kratochwill, T.R. 249
Kutnick, P. 117

Laban, R. 12, 28, 30, 69
Laffoon, D. 101
Lahad, M. 87, 89, 94
Landa, R. 191–2
Landreth, G. 199
Laub, D. 147–8
Laurie, S. 246
Laverty, S. 233
Leite, T. 130, 140
Levinge, A. 232

Levy, F.J. 28–31
Lewis, D. 32
Lewis, J. 247
Lewis, L. 101
Lincoln, Y. 260
Lindkvist, M. 201
Linesch, D.G. 64, 68, 72, 76
Lloyd, B. 146, 172
Lög um grunnskóla 146
Loman, S. 180, 186, 192, 199, 214
Lorden, S. 246, 254–5
Lord, S. 199, 209
Lotan, M. 248
Lowe, M. 220
Low, K.G. 64, 68, 72, 77
Lyshak-Stelzer, F. 147

McArdle, P. 63, 64, 68, 72, 76, 116, 121
MacBeath, J. 115, 117
McFarlane, P. 16
McFerran, K. 259–60
McLean, J.E. 263
McLeod, J. 102–3, 233
McNiff, S. 14
McQueen, C. 64
Mahony, J. 165
Main, M. 32
Malchiodi, C.A. 146, 149
Marcus, D. 211
Marcus, D. 199
Martinsone, K. 13
Matthews, J. 167, 173
Meadows, A. 261
Meek, M. 246–7
Meekums, B. 233
Meltzer, D. 218
Meltzer, H. 120
Merker, B. 243
Merriam, S. 33
Meyer, M.A. 146, 147
Meyerowitz-Katz, J. 167, 218
Miller, S. 201–2
Mills, J.C. 86
Min, Y. 95
Mitrani, J. 193
Mittledorf, W. 199
Mochizuki, A. 246, 254
Mohatt, G. 33
Monsegur, T. 188
Montague, J. 247
Moreno, J. 121
Moreno, Z. 121
Moringhaus, K. 64
Moriya, D. 16, 149
Moser, P. 149
Murray, L. 60, 70

National Autistic Society 217, 232
National Literacy Trust 85
National Statistics Office 85, 88

National Union of Teachers (NUT) 13
Nazarova, N. 13
Nicholas, J. 265
NIMH 179
Nind, M. 263, 268
Noble, J. 198–200, 205, 210
Nordoff, P. 64, 138, 232
Nozaki, K. 246, 254

Oaklander, V. 86
O'Brien, F. 146, 162
Ockleford, A. 130, 261
Odom, S. 260, 262
Office for National Statistics 59–60, 71
Ofsted 60, 115, 117
Ogletree, B. 263
O'Keefe, D.J. 117
Oldfield, A. 232, 237
Olley, J. 204
Olweus, D. 43–4
O'Neill, M. 181–2, 182
Osborne, J. 60
Ottarsdottir, U. 146

Parteli, L. 199
Paternite, C.E. 60
Patey-Tyler, H. 232
Patterson, Z. 218
Patton, G. 117, 118
Pavlicevic, M. 204, 233
Payne, H. 10–11, 64, 68, 72
Pennell, D. 246
Perason, A. 115
Perera, R. 116
Perry, M. 261
Peter, M. 11
Peterson, A. 116
Pifalo, T. 147
Pitkin, S.E. 246, 254–5
Pleasant-Metcalf, A.M. 149
Podell, D. 147–8
Porrino, L. 61
Pretchtl, H. 246
Prifitera, A. 150, 156–7
Primavera, L. 182
Primus, P. 45
Probst, W. 130
Prokofiev, F. 167

Quibell, T. 116, 124–5

Raghavendra, P. 259
Rankin, A.B. 148
Rapoport, J. 61
Read Johnson, D. 101, 106, 108, 111
Reid, S. 199, 211, 214
Renwick, F. 86, 95
Riley, S. 64, 68, 72, 76
Ritter, M. 64, 68, 72, 77
Robarts, J. 199, 232
Robbins, C. 64, 232
Robertson, J. 129, 131–3
Robson, C. 102
Rogers, C. 89, 101, 274
Rollins, P.R. 265
Romski, M. 254
Rose, G. 165
Rothwell, N. 98
Rowing, L. 60, 70, 70–1
Rubin, C. 248
Rubin, J.A. 146–7
Ryan, V. 199

Saklofske, D. 150, 156–7
Sandel, S. 45, 186, 192
Sanderson, P. 10–14, 63–4, 70, 220
Savoye, C. 44
Schalkwijk, F.W. 130
Schanin, M. 254
Schaverien, J. 164
Schlosser, R.W. 259–60, 260
Schmais, D. 67–9, 184, 192
Schopler, E. 204
Schore, A. 161
Scott, F. 219
Scottish Executive 59, 130
Scottish Parliament 129
Secondary SEAL 116
Selekman, M. 98–100
Sevcik, R. 254
Shalem, O. 254
Shapiro, D.A. 203
Sherborne, V. 20, 68–9, 200, 205–6, 208–9, 212–13
Siegel-Causey, E. 243–5
Siegel, E. 184
Sigafoos, J. 245–6, 253, 260, 263, 268
Silverman, D. 221
Simon, R. 167
Slaby, R.G. 44–5, 55
Spalding, B. 86, 95
Stake, R. 186
Stein-Safran, D. 16
Stephenson, J. 259–61
Stern, D. 185, 199, 204, 208, 212–13, 214, 224, 247
Stinson, S.W. 28, 31
Stoll, L. 117
Strauss, A. 150
Stronach-Buschel, B. 146
Subirana, V. 180
Surat, M.M. 50
Surrey, J. 29

Talwar, S. 146
Thomas, R. 116
Tiegerman, E. 182
Tinbergen, E.A. 218
Tinbergen, N. 218
Tortora, S. 28–33, 180, 193
Trevarthen, C. 180–3, 197–8, 204, 207, 214, 245–6
Troutman, A.C. 260
Turry, A. 211
Tustin, F. 218

Valente, L. 11
Van der Wijk, J.-B. 99, 109
Villena Fresquet, O. 187, 190–1
Viloca, L. 180, 190
Voracek, M. 214, 260–1
Vygotsky, L.S. 199

Wadsworth-Hervey, L. 15
Wahlstrom, J. 246–7
Wallace, J. 149
Waller, D. 10, 13, 64, 149
Warden, D. 117
Warwick, A. 11, 232, 235–6
Welch, G. 130
Wells, A.M. 61, 67
Wells, J. 61, 79
Welsby, C. 149
Wendt, O. 260
Wengrower, H. 11, 29, 149, 180–1, 188
Wesecky, A. 247
Westling, D. 260–1, 263
Wetherby, A.M. 263
Wethered, A.G. 200
White, E. 186
Whittaker, J.B. 44, 46–53, 55–6
WHO/UNESCO/UNICEF 117
Wieder, S. 180, 198–202, 210
Wigram, T. 10, 15, 214, 232, 243, 247–8, 252, 260–1, 264, 268
Wildsmith, B. 49
Williams, D. 198, 206–7
Williamson, G.G. 32
Wilson, B.L. 130
Wilson, C. 247
Wing, L. 218, 231
Winn, L. 100, 109
Winnicott, D.W. 30, 62, 64, 68, 188, 192–3, 219–20, 228
Witt-Engerstrom, I. 243, 246
Wittaker, J.W.B. 29
Woddis, J. 149
Woodward, A. 199, 232
Woodward, S. 130, 138
Wosch, T. 268

Yalom, I.D. 63, 67, 76
Yin, R.K. 88, 102, 104, 150, 186, 203, 233

Zeedyk, M. 181–2
Zimmermann, S. 130